Treating Addiction from an Islāmic Psychology Perspective

This book provides an understanding of behavioural and substance disorders from an Islāmic psychology perspective.

Despite the religious prohibitions against the use of most substances, addiction is a significant psychosocial and spiritual problem both in Muslim majority countries and among Muslim minorities. However, many Muslim with substance use disorder have been left to suffer in silence because addictive behaviours are considered taboo. Not only do feelings of guilt, shame, and a fear of being stigmatised and excluded from community prevent many from seeking therapeutic and spiritual interventions, there are also limited culturally sensitive service provisions offering help for Muslims with addictive behaviours. This book will synthesise the body of knowledge of the psychology of addiction from an Islāmic perspectives to foster awareness and understanding of addictive behaviours to break that stigma. It will also provide knowledge required to respond effectively to Muslim clients that psychotherapists and counsellors might encounter in their clinical practice, presenting a step-by-step application of Rassool's Islāmic Psychotherapy Practice model in working with clients with addictive behaviours.

This book will be a valuable read for Islāmic psychologists, psychotherapists, and counsellors, addiction researchers and specialists, and students in these fields.

G. Hussein Rassool is a professor of Islāmic Psychology at the Centre for Islāmic Studies and Civilisations, Charles Sturt University, Australia and Director of Studies, Department of Islāmic Psychology, Psychotherapy and Counselling, Al Balagh Academy. In addition, he is Chair of Al Balagh Institute of Islāmic Psychology Research. He is a fellow of the Royal Society of Public Health (FRSPH), the International Association of Islāmic Psychology (FIAIP), and a Trustee Board Member of the International Association of Muslim Psychologists. He is a member of the International Society of Substance Use Professionals (MISSUP).

Focus Series on Islāmic Psychology and Psychotherapy
Series Editor: Professor Dr. G. Hussein Rassool, Professor
of Islāmic Psychology

About the Series

In contemporary times, there is increasing focus on the need to adapt
approaches of psychology, counselling psychology and psychotherapy to
accommodate the integration of spirituality and psychology. With the
increasing focus on the need to meet the wholistic needs of Muslims, there
was a call to adapt approaches to the understanding of behaviour and experiences from an Islāmic epistemological and ontological worldview.

The aim of the Focus Series on Islāmic psychology and psychotherapy
is to introduce a range of educational, clinical and research interventions
relating to Islāmic psychology and psychotherapy that are authentic,
practical, concise, and based on cutting-edge research. Each volume
focuses on a particular aspect of Islāmic psychology and psychotherapy,
its application with a specific client group, a particular methodology or
approach, or a critical analysis of existing and emergent theoretical and
historical ideas.

Each book in the Focus Series is written, in accessible language, with
the assumption that the readers have no prior knowledge of Islāmic psychology and psychotherapy.

Maristāns and Islāmic Psychology
A Historical Model for Modern Implementation
Rania Awaad and Merve Nursoy-Demir

Treating Addiction from an Islāmic Psychology Perspective
By G. Hussein Rassool

**Spiritual Integration in Islāmic Psychotherapy: Unveiling the
Therapist's Soul**
By G. Hussein Rassool

Treating Addiction from an Islāmic Psychology Perspective

G. Hussein Rassool

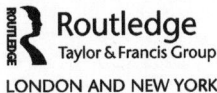
Routledge
Taylor & Francis Group

LONDON AND NEW YORK

First published 2025
by Routledge
4 Park Square, Milton Park, Abingdon, Oxon OX14 4RN

and by Routledge
605 Third Avenue, New York, NY 10158

Routledge is an imprint of the Taylor & Francis Group, an informa business

British Library Cataloguing-in-Publication Data
A catalogue record for this book is available from the British Library

ISBN: 978-1-032-66448-4 (hbk)
ISBN: 978-1-032-66916-8 (pbk)
ISBN: 978-1-032-66921-2 (ebk)

DOI: 10.4324/9781032669212

Typeset in Times New Roman
by SPi Technologies India Pvt Ltd (Straive)

Dedicated to Asiyah Maryam bint Adam Ibn Hussein Ibn Hassim Ibn Sahaduth Ibn Rosool Ibn Olee Al Mauritiusy, Isra Oya, Idrees Khattab, Adam Ali Hussein, Reshad Hassan, Yasmin Soraya, BeeBee Mariam, Bibi Safian & Hassim, Dr Najmul Hussein, and Mohammed Ali.

Abu Hurayrah reported the Prophet Muhammad (ﷺ) as saying: "If anyone pursues a path in search of knowledge, Allāh will thereby make easy for him a path to paradise; and he who is made slow by his actions will not be speeded by his genealogy." (Sunan Abū Dāwūd)

Contents

Illustrations

Figures

Tables

Preface

Addiction, although a universal phenomenon, has received relatively little attention from an Islāmic standpoint despite its significant physical, psycho-social, and spiritual impact on the individuals. The misuse of various substances like nicotine, alcohol, prescription medications, over-the-counter drugs, illicit substances, and gambling has risen sharply in recent years, contributing to health and socio-economic challenges. However, limited epidemiological studies in Muslim-majority countries make it challenging to ascertain the prevalence of pharmacological and non-pharmacological addictions among Muslim communities. Additionally, determining the prevalence of alcohol and substance use disorder and gambling among Muslims is hindered by the stigma associated with reporting such behaviours. Despite religious prohibitions, Muslims have been affected by the use of alcohol, drugs, tobacco, and shisha smoking. Islām categorically prohibits the use of intoxicants and gambling, considering them as the "Mother of all evils."

The book *Treating Addiction from an Islāmic Psychology Perspective* addresses the pressing need for understanding addictive behaviours from an Islāmic perspective within the context of Islāmic psychology. It aims to synthesise existing knowledge on the psychology of addiction with Islāmic principles, catering to health and social care professionals who encounter Muslim clients with addictive behaviours. As the field of Islāmic psychology continues to evolve, there is a pressing need to explore how Islāmic principles can inform our understanding and approach to addiction. Chapter 1, "Addictive behaviours: Introduction and context," sets the stage by examining the multifaceted nature of addiction. It explores concepts such as addiction characteristics, addictive experiences, cycles of addiction, theories of addiction, and the rise of new psychoactive substances. This chapter lays the groundwork for exploring Islāmic perspectives on addiction. Chapter 2, "Tracing the footsteps of addictive behaviours in Islāmic history," takes readers on a historical journey, uncovering the roots of addictive behaviours in Islāmic societies. It particularly examines the historical development of addiction concerning alcohol, drugs, caffeine, and gambling, providing valuable insights into evolving attitudes and approaches. Chapter 3, "Prohibitions and regulations regarding drugs, alcohol, and gambling: An Islāmic perspective," explores Qur'ânic injunctions and prophetic traditions that explicitly prohibit intoxicants and gambling. It examines the ethical and moral dimensions of these prohibitions and their implications for individuals and communities. Chapter 4, "Therapeutic psychosocial and pharmacological interventions," provides an overview of therapeutic approaches to addiction, including psychosocial interventions and pharmacological treatments. It integrates contemporary research with Islāmic ethics to address the unique needs of Muslim individuals seeking recovery. Chapter 5, "Faith-based solutions for addiction prevention in public health," examines the role of faith-based approaches in preventing addiction and promoting public health through an Islāmic lens. It highlights the intersection of faith and health promotion strategies. Chapter 6, "*Tawbah* (repentance) in addiction recovery: Understanding the process of change," explores the concept of *tawbah*, or repentance, as a central tenet of Islāmic spirituality and personal transformation. It examines how *tawbah* can facilitate healing and recovery from addiction. Chapter 7, "Spiritual healing: An Islāmic perspective on addressing addiction," focuses on the role of spirituality in addiction recovery, drawing on Islāmic teachings and practices to offer guidance and support. It also explores spiritual capital in addiction recovery and principles of Islāmic therapeutic interventions.

Through these chapters, the book provides a comprehensive understanding of addiction within Islāmic contexts, offering insights into historical, religious, and therapeutic perspectives. This book aims to bridge the gap between the psychology of addiction and Islāmic teachings, offering insights, guidance, and therapeutic interventions for therapists, counsellors, mental health practitioners, and clinical psychologists navigating the complexities of addiction within Islāmic communities.

Acknowledgements

All Praise is due to Allāh and may the peace and blessings of Allāh be upon our Prophet Muhammad (ﷺ), his family and his companions.

I extend my heartfelt thanks to Grace McDonnell, Editor at Routledge, for her invaluable suggestions and guidance throughout the development of the book's proposal. Her constructive feedback has been instrumental in shaping the content and direction of this book. I would also like to express my gratitude to Prisha Revar, Editorial Assistant at Routledge, for her unwavering support and assistance throughout this endeavour. I would like to acknowledge the support and encouragement of my colleagues at the Centre for Islāmic Studies & Civilisations, Charles Sturt University, Australia. In particular, I extend my sincere appreciation to Dr. Zuleyha Keskin, Associate Head of School at the Centre for Islāmic Studies and Civilizations, for her support. I express my gratitude to the past and current students of Islāmic Counselling and Psychology (Level 2), Addiction Counselling and Islāmic psychology, Islāmic Marriage Counselling, and Mental Health, *Jinn* Possession and Islāmic Psychology, Child Psychology: Western Insights and Islāmīc Perspectives at Al-Balagh Academy for the invaluable lessons and insights they have provided me throughout my journey in this field. Their dedication and commitment to learning and exploring the anatomy of Islāmic psychotherapy and counselling have been instrumental in shaping my knowledge and skills in this domain.

I am incredibly grateful to my beloved parents, who instilled in me the importance of education. Their unwavering love and guidance have been instrumental in shaping who I am today, and I am truly grateful for their wisdom and encouragement. I am humbled and deeply grateful for the unwavering love and support of Mariam, Idrees Khattab Ibn Adam Ali Hussein Ibn Hussein Ibn Hassim Ibn Sahaduth Ibn Rosool Al Mauritiusy, Adam Ali Hussein, Reshad Hasan, Yasmin Soraya, Isra Oya, Asiyah Maryam, Nabila Akhrif, Nusaybah Burke, Musa Burke, Fatima Azzahra, Dr. Najmul Hussein, and Mohammed Ali. Their presence in my life is a blessing, and I am forever indebted to them for their love, support, and inspiration.

I am grateful to acknowledge the invaluable contributions of my teachers, who have played a crucial role in enabling me to deepen my understanding of authentic Islām. Through their guidance and teachings, I have been able to embark on the right path, following the Creed of *Ahlus-Sunnah wa'l-Jamaa'ah*. I sincerely pray to Allāh that He forgives me and accepts my humble effort in writing this book. May He make it a source of benefit and fruitfulness for all those who find it useful and informative. May this book serve as a means of guidance and understanding for those who seek knowledge and insight. Finally, whatever benefits and correctness you find within this book are out of the Grace of Allāh, Alone, and whatever mistakes you find are mine alone. I pray to Allāh to forgive me for any unintentional shortcomings regarding the contents of this book and to make this humble effort helpful and fruitful to any interested parties.

مَّآ أَصَابَكَ مِنْ حَسَنَةٍ فَمِنَ ٱللَّهِ وَمَآ أَصَابَكَ مِن سَيِّئَةٍ فَمِن نَّفْسِكَ

- *Whatever of good befalls you, it is from Allāh; and whatever of ill befalls you, it is from yourself.*

(An-Nisā' 4:79, interpretation of the meaning)

Praise be to Allāh, we seek His help and His forgiveness. We seek refuge with Allāh from the evil of our own souls and from our bad deeds. Whomsoever Allāh guides will never be led astray, and whomsoever Allāh leaves astray, no one can guide. I bear witness that there is no god but Allāh, and I bear witness that Muhammad is His slave and Messenger (*Sunan al-Nasa'i: Kitaab al-Jumu'ah, Baab kayfiyyah al-khutbah*).

- Fear Allāh as He should be feared and die not except in a state of Islām (as Muslims) with complete submission to Allāh (Ali-'Imran 3:102, interpretation of the meaning).[1]
- O mankind! Be dutiful to your Lord, Who created you from a single person, and from him He created his wife, and from them both He created many men and women, and fear Allāh through Whom you demand your mutual (rights), and (do not cut the relations of) the wombs (kinship) Surely, Allāh is Ever an All-Watcher over you) (Al-Nisā' 4:1, interpretation of the meaning).
- O you who believe! Keep your duty to Allāh and fear Him and speak (always) the truth) (Al-Ahzāb 33:70, interpretation of the meaning).
- What comes to you of good is from Allāh, but what comes to you of evil, [O man], is from yourself (An-Nisā 4:79, interpretation of the meaning).

The essence of this book is based on the following notions:

- The fundamental of as a religion is based on the Oneness of God.
- The source of knowledge is based on the Qur'ān and Hadīth (*Ahl as-Sunnah wa'l-Jamā'ah*).
- Empirical knowledge from sense perception is also a source of knowledge through the work of classical and contemporary Islāmic scholars and research.
- Islām takes a holistic approach to health: physical, psychological, social, emotional, and spiritual health cannot be separated.
- Muslims have an Islāmic or Qur'ânic worldview different from the Western-oriented worldview.
- It is a sign of respect that Muslims would utter or repeat the words "Peace and Blessing Be Upon Him" after hearing (or writing) the name of Prophet Muhammad (ﷺ).

Note

1 The translations of the meanings of the verses of the Qur'ān in this book have been taken, with some changes, from Saheeh International, The Qur'ān: Arabic Text with corresponding English meanings.

1 Addictive behaviours

Introduction and context

Introduction

Globally, addictive behaviours are now regarded as part of the fabric of society and are considered as a public health problem. In the above Qur'ânic verse addressed to believers, it counsels individuals to refrain from participating in specific activities considered harmful and linked to the influence of *shaytān* (satan). The focus of the prohibited actions includes the consumption of intoxicants and participation in gambling. Islām discourages these practices due to their potential harm to individuals both physically and spiritually. The fundamental message is to avoid engaging in these activities to guarantee success, as they are viewed as transgressions that could divert believers from the path of righteousness and exclusive devotion to Allāh (God). The term *mudmin* was employed by Ibn al-Qayyim (2010) refers to a person habitually engaged with something, similar to what we understand as addiction today. In classical contexts, it described someone habitually involved with a particular substance or behaviour. It was narrated from Abu Hurayrah (may Allāh be pleased with him) that the Messenger of Allāh (ﷺ) said: "The one who is addicted to wine is like one who worships idols." (Ibn Majah). The comparison between someone addicted to wine and a worshiper of idols highlights the severity of the addiction in Islāmic teachings. Just as worshipping idols is considered a grave sin due to its deviation from monotheistic principles, addiction to wine or any intoxicant is viewed as a serious transgression against oneself and one's faith. However, Abdul-Rahman (2023) emphasises that in these narratives, the term "*mudmin*" was employed to broadly characterise intentional and habitual engagement with something, rather than specifically denoting psychological addiction as it is understood in contemporary contexts.

The societal fabric exhibits a natural inclination towards both pharmacological and non-pharmacological addictive behaviours, including a preference for alcohol consumption ("our favourite drug"), tobacco, illicit drugs and the misuse of prescription painkillers, and emerging synthetic

DOI: 10.4324/9781032669212-1

drugs. Additionally, participation in non-pharmacological addictive behaviours like gambling, cyber addiction, eating disorders, and Internet addiction is prevalent. This complex interconnection between substance misuse and various behavioural dependencies reflects a broad spectrum of addictive tendencies (Rassool, 2011, 2020). The increased use of medically prescribed psychoactive substances, such as antidepressants, painkillers, and sleeping tablets, has heightened the risk of individuals misusing these medications, contributing significantly to the prevalence of iatrogenic addiction (referring to drug addiction or misuse stemming from medical treatment) (Rassool, 2011, 2020). Addictive behaviours transcend demographic differences and impact individuals irrespective of age, gender, race, marital status, residence, income, or lifestyle. The implications of alcohol and substance use disorder extend beyond individual users to encompass families, communities, and society at large. Despite global efforts, including initiatives like the "war on drugs," legislative measures, punitive actions, health promotion, and treatment programmes, many countries struggle to effectively address addiction (Rassool, 2021). Traditional approaches, such as abstinence-oriented strategies, have often failed to fully eradicate various forms of addiction. In contrast to abstinence-focused cultures, some countries have adopted a harm-reduction approach to manage addictive behaviours. This strategy, which diverges from prevailing abstinence-based and zero-tolerance methods, is particularly absent in Muslim-majority countries.

Islāmic principles have long advocated restrictions on the use of harmful substances, effectively limiting their prevalence within Muslim communities. It is important to highlight that the Islāmic perspective on the "War on Drugs" traces back to the 14th century. Despite Islāmic prohibitions on addictive substances and activities, Muslim communities are not immune to issues such as alcohol, drug, tobacco, gambling, eating disorders, and cybersex addiction. A significant concern within Muslim communities is the reluctance of addicted individuals to seek help or access treatment services due to feelings of guilt, shame, fear of stigma, and potential exclusion from family and community life. Limited culturally sensitive services further compound the difficulty for Muslims-seeking assistance with addictive behaviours (Rassool, 2011, 2020). Addressing addiction in the Muslim community requires a holistic approach, encompassing preventive health education, detoxification, harm reduction, psychosocial support, education, and spiritual interventions. It's noted that for a more comprehensive understanding of addictive behaviours, readers are encouraged to refer to Rassool (2011, 2021), as the scope of this chapter does not allow for an in-depth exploration of the topic. The aims of this chapter are to provide an overview of the concept of addiction and the common characteristics of addictive behaviours. The chapter also focuses on the cycles and stages of addiction and the nature of addiction in Muslims communities.

What is addiction?

Addiction refers to individuals experiencing a compulsion and dependence on either a psychoactive substance like alcohol or drugs or a particular behaviour such as gambling, sex, or physical activity. Essentially, addictive behaviour is an explanation for why individuals engage in certain actions and persist in maintaining those behaviours despite facing adverse consequences. A comprehensive definition of addiction from the American Society of Addiction Medicine (ASAM) (2011) is that

> Addiction is a primary, chronic disease of brain reward, motivation, memory and related circuitry. Addiction affects neurotransmission and interactions within reward structures of the brain, including the nucleus accumbens, anterior cingulate cortex, basal forebrain and amygdala, such that motivational hierarchies are altered and addictive behaviours, which may or may not include alcohol and other drug use, supplant healthy, self-care related behaviours. Addiction also affects neurotransmission and interactions between cortical and hippocampal circuits and brain reward structures, such that the memory of previous exposures to rewards (such as food, sex, alcohol and other drugs) leads to a biological and behavioural response to external cues, in turn triggering craving and/or engagement in addictive behaviours.

The above definition takes a neurobiological orientation of addiction emphasising its status as a primary and chronic disease affecting various brain functions, particularly the reward system. This perspective highlights the intricate and complex nature of addictive behaviours, emphasising their biological and behavioural components and their impact on decision-making and lifestyle choices. The American Psychological Association (2024) defines addiction as a condition marked by psychological and/or physical dependence on substances like drugs or alcohol, as well as on activities or behaviours. This definition highlights the broad spectrum of addictive experiences, including not only substances like drugs and alcohol but also various activities or behaviours. The concept of addiction (Rassool, 2020) has been modified and viewed as

> a relapsing disorder with both neuro-pharmacological and behavioural components. It manifests in various forms, including those linked to pharmacological substances like tobacco, drugs, or alcohol, as well as behaviours such as gambling, overeating, sexual addiction,

and, notably, excessive social media use. The disorder may involve physical or psychological dependence, or a combination of both, and is characterised by cravings and dependence.

(p. 66)

This comprehensive definition captures the essence of addiction by acknowledging the diverse manifestations of addiction, encompassing both substance-related and behavioural dependence, while emphasising the relapsing nature of the disorder.

Classifications and diagnostic criteria

In the United States, the term "addiction" is often used interchangeably with substance use disorder or substance dependence. In the British context, the equivalent terms are "substance misuse" or "drug and alcohol misuse." This highlights the linguistic variations in expressing the concept of problematic substance use between the two regions. The Diagnostic and Statistical Manual of Mental Disorders (DSM-5) (American Psychiatric Association, 2013) does not specifically define "addiction." Instead, it combines the DSM-IV categories of substance abuse and substance dependence into a single continuum disorder called substance use disorder. This disorder is assessed on a spectrum ranging from mild to severe. In DSM-5, the only addictive disorder listed as a diagnosable condition under a new category of behavioural addictions is gambling disorder. Internet gaming disorder and caffeine use disorder are included in Section III of the manual, indicating they need further research before being considered formal disorders. Notably, Internet sex addiction or cybersex addiction is not included in the DSM-5 manual.

Brief overview of the theories of addiction

Various models and theories attempt to explain alcohol and drug use, ranging from genetic and biological causes to social or psychological factors. The bio-psychosocial model views addiction as both a physiological and a psycho-social phenomenon, while certain models highlight a psycho-spiritual cause. Reasons for initiating substance use may differ from those for continued use, illustrating the multifaceted nature of addiction causation. Theories can be categorised into moral, disease, psychological, sociocultural, genetic/neuropharmacological, bio-psychosocial, and spiritual perspectives (Rassool, 2021). West (2006) examines approximately 30 theories regarding addiction's origin, spanning from rational choice to cognitive, behavioural, and economic features, including operant learning and classical conditioning, and the role of neurotransmitters like dopamine. This comprehensive exploration reflects addiction's multi-faceted nature, incorporating diverse perspectives and contributing to our understanding of its origins.

The moral perspective attributes addiction to moral weakness, bad character, or a weak will, emphasising individual responsibility and deviation from accepted norms. This approach lacks recognition of a biological basis for addiction and tends to employ a "victim-blaming" approach, focusing on behavioural control through social disapproval, spiritual guidance, moral persuasion, or imprisonment. In contrast, the disease perspective views addiction as linked to genetic or biological factors, adopting the sick-role concept. It sees addiction as a unique, irreversible, and progressive disease, highlighting the individual's inability to control consumption and advocating abstinence as the primary option for management. This concept is fundamental to the philosophy of alcoholics anonymous (AA), narcotics anonymous (NA), and gamblers anonymous (GA).

The genetic/neuropharmacological theory suggests that addiction may result from genetic or induced biological abnormalities. Family studies, such as those by Merikangas et al. (1998), show a clustering of alcohol use disorders within families, indicating a genetic predisposition to addiction. Cumulative evidence, as highlighted by Agrawal and Lynskey (2008) and Prescott et al. (2016), strongly suggests a significant genetic contribution to addiction vulnerability, particularly concerning substances like alcohol, tobacco, and illicit drugs. Moreover, genetic factors contribute to the co-occurrence or comorbidity of addiction with other psychiatric disorders. Studies, like Müller and Homberg (2015), examining the role of serotonin (5-HT) system in addiction pathways associated with various substances, emphasise its significant contribution. Additionally, neurotransmitters like norepinephrine, as discussed by Foster and Weinshenker (2019), may also play a role in addiction.

The psychoanalytic theory of addiction attributes addictive behaviours to fixation during psychosexual development or as manifestations of unconscious death wishes, often conceptualised as a form of "slow suicide." This theory involves conflicts between repressed ideas and defence mechanisms against them, along with a deficient ego (Leeds & Morgenstern, 1996). In contrast, behavioural theories view addiction as learned behaviour through classical and operant conditioning. Specific factors associated with substances may drive the desire to use drugs, with positive reinforcement playing a significant role due to the pleasurable sensations induced by drugs. Continued substance use is reinforced by the pursuit of pleasure or, in some cases, the fear of withdrawal. Cue exposure theory, rooted in classical conditioning, posits that cues play a crucial role in the development and maintenance of addictive behaviour (Drummond et al., 1995). The personality theory of addiction emphasises the role of individual traits and characteristics in the development and persistence of addictive behaviours, challenging the notion of an "addictive personality." While addiction predisposition involves bio-psychosocial factors, traits such as hyperactivity, sensation-seeking, antisocial behaviour, and impulsivity have been associated with substance use (Sher et al., 1991).

Social learning theory stresses cognitive processes in understanding the effects of alcohol or drugs, emphasising the role of role modelling and the need to conform in forming and maintaining addictive behaviours. Orford's (2001) theory of "Excessive Appetites" extends this perspective, suggesting that an individual's involvement with "appetitive activities" is influenced by biological, personality, social, and ecological determinants. This highlights the multifaceted nature of personality traits and social influences in addiction. Sociocultural theories of addiction encompass various sub-theories such as systems theory, anomie theory, family interaction theory, anthropological theory, economic theory, gateway theory, and availability theory. Addiction, from a sociological perspective, is viewed as individual behaviour with social implications, affecting others and subject to societal control (Adiran, 2003). The cultural model recognises cultural and religious attitudes as protective factors against alcohol and drug addiction, with ethnicity and religious values strongly influencing drug-taking and drinking behaviour (Oyefeso et al., 2000). Sociocultural factors impacting drug and alcohol use include gender, age, occupation, social class, ethno-cultural background, subcultures, alienated groups, family dysfunction, and religious affiliation. The biopsychosocial model (Engel, 1977) incorporates not only biological factors but also psychological and social aspects that influence health and disease. This model has been revitalised to take into account the personal, interpersonal relations, and institutional factors in relation to health and disease (Bolton, 2023). Additionally, the spiritual dimension is suggested as an additional component in the bio-psychosocial theory (Hamond & Rassool, 2006). This underlines the broad range of sociocultural factors influencing addiction, emphasising the interconnectedness of biological, psychological, social, environmental, and spiritual dimensions.

Professor Malik Badri (2009) did not introduce a specific model of addiction but expressed critique towards liberal attitudes on sex in the West, linking them to the surge in drug addiction and the AIDS crisis. He argued that the language used to discuss drug use in the West has contributed to a permissive atmosphere for alcohol and drug misuse. In opposition to Western perspectives, he rejected a non-judgemental stance and urged against the acceptance of promiscuity and substance use. Badri called for a paradigm shift based on Islāmic principles, advocating for a morally grounded approach to addressing addiction. He asserted that Islām's overarching purpose is to intervene in human affairs for societal betterment, presenting an alternative viewpoint challenging Western paradigms of addiction treatment.

Common characteristics of addictive behaviours

The common characteristics associated with addictive behaviours include intense obsession, continued engagement despite causing harm, compulsive involvement, withdrawal symptoms upon cessation, loss of control, denial of the severity, efforts to hide the behaviour, episodes of blackout, the presence of depression, and low self-esteem (Engs, 1987). Table 1.1 presents a summary of the characteristics of addictive behaviours.

Some individuals may experience episodes of memory loss or amnesia related to the addictive activity (alcohol) and low-self-esteem and

Table 1.1 Characteristics of addictive behaviours

Characteristics	Explanations
Preoccupation with the addiction	Excess amount of time and energy is spent thinking about, obtaining, and engaging in the addictive behaviour.
Loss of interest in other activities	Addictive behaviour becomes the primary focus, and other aspects of life become less important.
Negative impact on responsibilities	Addiction tends to interfere with daily responsibilities, such as work, school, or family obligations. Neglect important tasks or relationships in favour of the addictive activities.
Loss of control	Struggle to control their behaviour despite negative consequences. Find it challenging to limit or stop their engagement in the addictive behaviour or substance use.
Denial	Exhibit denial about the extent of their problem. Minimise the negative consequences or rationalise their behaviour, Difficult for them to recognise the need for intervention.
Continued use despite harm	When faced with adverse consequences, individuals with addiction persist in their addictive behaviour. Include negative effects on physical health, social, psychological, spiritual, relationships, or professional life.
Tolerance	Require increasing amounts of the substance or more intense engagement in the behaviour to achieve the desired effect. Contribute to a cycle of escalating consumption or engagement.
Compulsive behaviour	Involves a compulsion to engage in the behaviour or use the substance, driven by intense cravings.
Withdrawal symptoms	When the addictive behaviour or substance use is reduced or discontinued, individuals may experience withdrawal symptoms. Symptoms can be physical, emotional, or psychological and often drive a compulsion to resume the addictive behaviour to alleviate the discomfort.
Cyclical nature	Follows a cyclical pattern of highs and lows. Periods of intense engagement in the addictive behaviour may be followed by remorse, attempts to quit, and then relapse.

depression. These features illustrate the persistent nature of addictive behaviours, encompassing cognitive, emotional, and behavioural aspects. It is important to note that these characteristics can manifest differently based on the specific addiction, and not all may be present in every case. Individual experiences with addiction can vary widely and may be influenced by various factors, including ethnicity, cultural background, and individual differences. Religiosity, cultural context, social norms, and the perception of addiction within specific communities can all play significant roles in shaping how individuals experience and cope with addictive behaviours.

Addictive experiences and cycles of addiction

The process of addiction is influenced by three key sets of interrelated factors: individual characteristics, pharmacological aspects, and the context or setting in which drug or alcohol consumption occurs. Individual traits, including biological makeup, personality, age, and tolerance, shape the drug experience. Additionally, one's knowledge, attitudes, and expectations about a substance contribute to the subjective effects. Pharmacological factors involve the chemical properties of drugs, their types, dosage, and administration routes, all of which determine their impact on the body. The context or setting, encompassing the physical environment, cultural influences, and legal frameworks, further influences the overall addictive experiences (Rassool, 2018). Furthermore, patterns of drug or alcohol use can vary over time, progressing through stages of experimentation, recreational, tolerance and dependence, addiction, craving, attempts to quit or cut back, and lapse and relapse. These stages are shaped by the interplay of individual characteristics, pharmacological properties, and contextual factors. The cycles of addictive behaviour are presented in Figure 1.1.

The progression of substance use typically begins with an experimental stage where individuals use psychoactive substances due to curiosity, anticipation of effects, and availability. There is no discernible usage pattern, and substance choice is often influenced by factors like availability, reputation, subculture, fashion, and peer-group influence. This phase carries a risk of infections, medical complications, or overdose, especially with practices like injecting or using adulterated substances. Subsequently, individuals may enter the recreational phase, where drug or alcohol consumption is primarily for pleasure and relaxation. Usage patterns are disciplined, often limited to specific occasions like weekends, with a preference for a particular substance (drug of choice). Substance use complements social and recreational activities, resulting in minimal adverse medical or social consequences. Ghaferi et al. (2016) identified evidence suggesting a progression from experimentation to dependence among some Muslim participants, highlighting potential vulnerabilities within

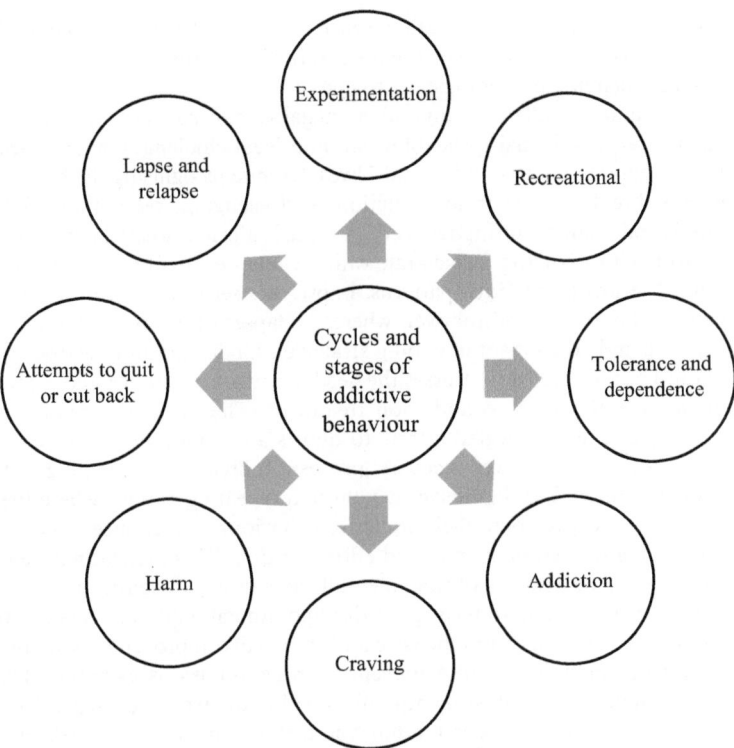

Figure 1.1 The cycles of addictive behaviours.

this community. In the dependent phase of substance use, individuals exhibit regular and problematic alcohol or drug use, potentially becoming polydrug users. Psychological and/or physical dependence emerges, leading to more frequent and less controlled patterns of use. The obsession with the substance or activity takes precedence over other interests, including work and relationships. Withdrawal symptoms may occur when not using the substance or engaging in the behaviour, with injecting drugs being common and posing risks of intoxication, infections, and other medical complications. In the advanced stage of addiction, individuals experience chaotic behaviour dominated by substance use or addictive behaviour, resulting in a loss of autonomy. Despite negative consequences such as health issues, strained relationships, financial troubles, and legal complications, individuals remain trapped in compulsive engagement. Intense cravings in addiction reflect powerful urges for the substance or behavioural activity, often linked to neurobiological changes in the brain affecting reward and motivation centres (Sinha, 2013). Environmental cues, stressors, or emotional triggers can further intensify cravings, creating a challenging psychological struggle.

Addiction results in a myriad of negative consequences across personal, social, spiritual, psychological, and legal challenges, highlighting its profound impact on individuals' lives. Despite recognising the harmful effects, breaking free from addiction is challenging, often marked by lapses and relapses during recovery. A lapse is a brief, isolated incident of returning to addictive behaviour, while a relapse involves a more prolonged return to previous patterns. Lapses are setbacks that individuals can quickly regain control over, whereas relapses offer opportunities for learning and adjustment in coping strategies. Understanding relapse as a natural part of recovery stresses the need for ongoing support and a comprehensive approach to addiction treatment. The cycle of attempts to quit, relapse, and repeated efforts to quit is a common and challenging aspect of the addiction recovery process. Individuals struggling with addiction often find themselves caught in a repeating pattern where they intently try to overcome their addictive behaviours, experience a setback (relapse), and then make renewed efforts to quit. This cyclical nature of recovery can be emotionally and mentally demanding, fostering a sense of hopelessness, leading to feelings of disappointment, guilt, and shame. To address this cycle, a comprehensive and supportive approach to addiction treatment, including relapse prevention programmes, is essential. This approach involves addressing not only the physical aspects of dependence or addiction but also understanding and tackling the psychological, emotional, and social factors contributing to the cycle. Providing effective coping mechanisms, ongoing support, and fostering a positive mindset are crucial elements in breaking the cycle of attempts, relapse, and renewed efforts, facilitating a more sustainable path toward recovery. The cyclical nature of attempting to quit, experiencing relapse, and making renewed efforts in addiction recovery varies among individuals due to personal factors, pharmacological properties of substances or behaviours, and environmental influences. Individuals may enter and exit these cycles at different stages, with re-entry possible at any point. This variability underlines the complexity of addiction and emphasises the need for tailor-made and flexible approaches to intervention strategies and support.

Methodology of drug use

Understanding addictive behaviours related to drug use involves considering routes of drug administration and associated rituals. Paraphernalia used in drug consumption, such as hypodermic syringes or smoking instruments, act as cues that can increase drug use. Drug absorption varies based on the route of administration, influencing the speed of physical and psychological effects. Common routes include oral administration through liquid or tablets, injection for faster impact, and smoking, particularly for substances like cannabis, crack cocaine, and heroin. The choice of administration affects the amount delivered to the brain, delivery and elimination rates, and intensity of drug effects. Complications of injection include trauma, infections, overdose, poisoning, thrombosis, and embolism. Recognising various routes of drug administration is crucial in understanding the addictive process and its connection to rituals surrounding drug use.

Groups of psychoactive substances

The term "psychoactive drug" refers to substances that, when ingested, alter an individual's mental processes, mood, cognition, or behaviour by affecting neurotransmitter activity in the brain. These drugs, also called psychotropic substances, encompass various classes such as depressants, stimulants, hallucinogens, dissociative anaesthetics, narcotic analgesics (opioids), inhalants, and cannabis. They can have therapeutic uses, recreational purposes, and, in some cases, potential for abuse and dependence. Additionally, synthetic drugs, known as designer drugs or new psychoactive substances (NPS), are chemically engineered compounds created to mimic traditional psychoactive substances' effects. Table 1.2 depicts the category of drugs.

Table 1.2 Categories of drugs

Categories	Effects	Examples
Opioids	Primarily interact with opioid receptors, leading to pain relief and, in some cases, euphoria.	Heroin, morphine, hydrocodone, opium, Vicodin, oxycontin, Percocet, fentanyl, and codeine.
Stimulants	Increase alertness, energy, and arousal.	Cocaine, methamphetamine, Ecstasy*, Adderall, Ritalin, Synthetic Marijuana, Khat, and Caffeine.
Depressants	Slow down brain activity and induce relaxation.	Benzodiazepines, Rohypnol, Barbiturates, Xanax, and Valium. Alcohol and tobacco.
Hallucinogens	Alter perception, mood, and consciousness, often leading to hallucinations.	LSD, peyote and MDMA (Ecstasy*), Psilocybin (Liberty cap mushrooms), *Amanita muscaria* (Fly agaric mushrooms), morning glory seeds.

(Continued)

Table 1.2 (Continued)

Categories	Effects	Examples
Dissociatives	Induce a sense of detachment from one's surroundings or reality.	Ketamine, dextromethorphan (DXM) (found in cough medicines) and phencyclidine (PCP).
Inhalants	Lead to mind-altering effects.	Fumes of markers, paint, paint thinner, gasoline and glue, nitrous oxide, aerosol sprays, and room deodorisers.
Cannabis	Producing effects such as relaxation and altered perception.	Marijuana leaves, Hashish, hash oil, and Cannabis-based medicines, such as Sativex.
New psychoactive substance	Synthetic cannabinoids: sprayed onto plant material and sold as herbal smoking blends. Synthetic cathinones: these substances are designed to replicate the effects of stimulants like amphetamines or ecstasy. Synthetic opioids: mimic the effects of opioids like heroin or prescription painkillers. Synthetic hallucinogens: these compounds are designed to mimic the effects of hallucinogenic drugs like LSD. Synthetic stimulants: produce stimulant effects similar to amphetamines or cocaine.	Synthetic cannabinoids: Clockwork Orange, Black Mamba, K2, spice, and Exodus Damnation.Synthetic cathinones: bath salts. methylenedioxypyrovalerone (MDPV), mephedrone, alpha-PVP (Flakka), ethylone, and butylone. Synthetic opioids: fentanyl analogs. Carfentanil, acetylfentanyl, furanylfentanyl, butyrfentanyl, and 4-fluorobutyrfentanyl. Synthetic hallucinogens: 25i-NBOMe, Bromo-Dragonfly, and the more ketamine-like methoxetamine. Stimulant-type drugs: BZP, mephedrone, MPDV, NRG-1, Benzo Fury, MDAI, and ethylphenidate. Downer'/tranquiliser-type drugs: etizolam, pyrazolam, and flubromazepam.

Source: Adapted from Rassool (2021).

* Ecstasy is considered as a stimulant and hallucinogens because of its compound.

New addictions: New dangers in the 21st Century

In the 21st century, the landscape of addiction has evolved with the emergence of new substances and behaviours, presenting significant dangers. Traditional drugs are often reformulated into "designer drugs" to bypass existing drug laws and regulations due to political and socio-economic conditions. Synthetic cannabinoids, designed to mimic THC's effects, are sprayed onto plant material and sold as herbal smoking blends. Synthetic cathinones, known as "Bath salts," can induce stimulant effects and are ingested, inhaled, or injected in crystalline powder form, leading to severe agitation, hallucinations, and delirium. Flakka, another synthetic cathinone, gained attention for its stimulant properties and reported cases of erratic and dangerous behaviour in users, including extreme agitation, psychosis, and violent actions. Kratom, a plant-based substance used as traditional medicine in Southeast Asia, has emerged as a popular new psychoactive substance (UNODC, 2018). Synthetic opioids, such as fentanyl, are extremely potent and pose a high risk of overdose due to respiratory depression, contributing to the opioid epidemic. Illicitly manufactured fentanyl is particularly problematic as it is often mixed with other drugs. Synthetic hallucinogens and stimulants sold on blotter paper or as "bath salts" can have unpredictable and dangerous effects, while the substitution of cocaine and Ecstasy with prescription drugs like Vicodin and OxyContin presents new challenges. Captagon tablets, a compound substance of amphetamine, have a substantial market in Middle Eastern countries. PCP (phencyclidine), a dissociative anaesthetic, can induce hallucinations, delirium, and aggressive behaviour, with chronic use associated with cognitive impairment and mental health issues. Each synthetic substance poses unique risks, contributing to the complexity of addiction in contemporary society and introducing challenges in addressing drug-related issues.

Contemporary societal changes have led to the emergence of new behavioural patterns characterised by compulsive and problematic behaviours, extending beyond substance use. The widespread availability of the Internet has facilitated the rise of online gambling and cybersex addiction, while the term "nomophobia" represents the fear of being without a mobile phone, highlighting anxiety related to constant connectivity. These behavioural shifts highlight the multifaceted challenges posed by evolving technologies and their impact on mental health. Addressing these issues requires a comprehensive understanding of the interplay between technology, behaviour, and psychological health, fostering strategies for responsible and balanced engagement in the digital age.

Categories of drugs: Over-the-counter drugs

Over-the-counter (OTC) drugs are medications that can be purchased without a prescription. Many OTC medicinal preparations, readily available in pharmacies or chemist shops without a prescription, are often purchased for their non-medical therapeutic effects. Some individuals may intentionally misuse OTC medications for their psychoactive or euphoric effects. Commonly abused OTC drugs include cough syrups containing dextromethorphan, which can produce hallucinogenic effects at high doses. Additionally, some OTC pain relievers, such as those containing codeine, may be abused for their analgesic properties. The misuse of OTC drugs can lead to various health risks, including overdose, organ damage, and addiction.

Alcohol

Alcohol, specifically ethyl alcohol or ethanol, is a colourless, flammable liquid with a distinct smell and taste. It acts as a depressant on the central nervous system and is absorbed in various parts of the digestive system, including the mouth, oesophagus, and stomach. Once absorbed, alcohol is transported to the liver for metabolism, where enzymes break it down into acetaldehyde and subsequently into acetic acid, carbon dioxide, and water. Individuals vary in alcohol absorption rates due to physiological differences, stomach contents, and contextual factors. The enzyme acetaldehyde dehydrogenase plays a crucial role in the breakdown process. Alcohol can affect nutrient absorption and contribute to malnutrition or vitamin deficiencies, especially in heavy drinkers. Women generally become more intoxicated than men with the same alcohol amount due to factors such as fat distribution, hormonal status, and contraceptive use. Initially, small amounts of alcohol induce relaxation, euphoria, and reduced inhibition. As consumption increases, cognitive, perceptual, and behavioural impairments emerge, including slurred speech, poor coordination, unsteady gait, nystagmus (uncontrolled eye movement), impaired judgement, insomnia, hangovers, and blackouts.

Alcohol use disorder leads to severe health issues including nerve damage (polyneuropathy), heart and muscle diseases, stomach inflammation (alcoholic gastritis), liver conditions, pancreatitis, birth defects (foetal alcohol syndrome), and various cancers. It also contributes to high blood pressure, strokes, neuropsychiatric disorders like epilepsy, diabetes mellitus, and depressive disorders. These consequences illustrate the multifaceted impact of alcohol misuse on different bodily systems. Heavy drinkers often exhibit poor eating habits, leading to inadequate nutrition and deficient in essential vitamins like thiamine, crucial for normal growth and functioning of the nervous, digestive, and cardiovascular systems. Alcohol's impact on the stomach lining further delays vitamin absorption. This nutritional deficiency, combined with alcohol dependence, contributes to various issues including peripheral neuropathies, "alcohol dementia," and physical, immunological, and psychological disorders. Wernicke's encephalopathy, resulting from alcohol-induced thiamine (Vitamin B1) deficiency, presents symptoms like ataxia, involuntary eye movements, drowsiness, and confusion. Diagnosis can be challenging due to elusive symptoms, but prompt treatment with high thiamine doses can reverse symptoms and prevent brain damage or death. If untreated or inadequately treated, Wernicke's encephalopathy, may progress to Korsakoff's psychosis, characterised by severe memory impairment, anterograde and retrograde amnesia, confabulation, and apathy. The severity of issues is linked to the degree of alcohol dependence, emphasising the importance of addressing nutritional deficiencies in heavy drinkers. For women, harmful drinking has been linked to menstrual disorders and fertility problems. Women appear more susceptible to alcohol's influence just before or during their menstrual cycle compared to other times in the cycle: These consequences underscore the wide-ranging impact of alcohol on both physical and mental health.

Muslim communities universally adhere to the prohibition of alcohol consumption, as dictated by the teachings of the Qur'ân and *hadīth*. This prohibition is rooted in verses highlighting alcohol's negative consequences, such as impaired judgement and conflicts. Alcohol misuse within Muslim families profoundly impacts children and spouses. Children of alcoholic parents face higher risks of psychological disorders, behavioural problems, and adverse developmental outcomes, potentially leading to lower self-esteem and anxiety in adulthood. Spouses experience negative emotions, exhaustion, and potential physical or mental disorders, alongside financial difficulties due to their partner alcohol's consumption. Co-dependency is common, perpetuating denial and conflict avoidance while attempting to control or cure the drinker. Alcohol's impact on Muslim families encompasses psychological, behavioural, and socioeconomic dimensions.

Gambling disorder

The legalisation of gambling over the past decade has raised significant concerns within public health policy, evolving into a prominent form of behavioural addiction with global reach. Even in Muslim societies, influenced by Western values and psychosocial factors, gambling has gained acceptance. Gambling disorder, characterised by continual engagement in gambling activities leading to functional difficulties or distress, is a growing concern. Compulsive gambling, a behavioural addiction, involves a compulsive urge to continue gambling despite evident harms or negative consequences. Studies have shown similarities between gambling disorder and compulsive gambling in diagnostic criteria, symptoms, genetic susceptibilities, comorbidity rates, and their connection to biological markers and cognitive impairments (APA, 2013; Petry et al., 2014; Rash et al., 2016).

Gambling disorder encompasses a complex interplay of determinants including biological, psychological, socio-cultural, and neurochemical factors. Neurobiological mechanisms, notably the role of Norepinephrine, link hormonal responses to stress with arousal and risk-taking in compulsive gamblers (Potenza, 2013). Family environment also plays a crucial role, with significant correlations found between adolescents with pathological gambling and parents with gambling problems (Gupta & Derevensky, 1998). Genetic factors, featured in twin studies, indicate a notable responsibility for high-action gambling in male twins (Winters & Rich, 1998). Stress, coping strategies, impulsivity, and antisocial behaviour are significant risk factors, exacerbated by the accessibility of online gaming through the Internet and mobile phones. Co-existing disorders like substance use disorder and psychiatric disorders are prevalent among problem gamblers, particularly showing a strong association between alcohol use and gambling. Unlike substance use disorder, problem gambling may not exhibit recognisable signs, and individuals often deny the issue both to themselves and others, projecting a sense of power, control, and competitiveness. While many individuals gamble recreationally, problems arise when it becomes uncontrollable, leading to psychological, social, and financial difficulties (Rassool, 2021).

Maysar, the Arabic term for gambling, covers a range of activities, including divination with divine arrows, backgammon, chess, and lotteries. Imam Malik (may Allāh be pleased with him) differentiated gambling into two categories: games of chance engaged in for entertainment purposes and those specifically involving gambling (cited in Siddiqi, 1981). Islāmic Law (*Shar'iah*) explicitly prohibits gambling (based on the guidance found in the Qur'ân and *hadīth*. The specific types of activities categorised as gambling include the National Lottery Draw, scratch cards, football pools, bingo, slot machines, horse and dog races, betting with a bookmaker, online betting with a bookmaker on any event or sport, online gambling, games in a casino, and private betting (e.g., with friends or colleagues). This prohibition reflects the Islāmic principle of safeguarding individuals and society from the potential harms associated with gambling, aligning with broader ethical and social considerations within the Islāmic legal framework.

Internet and social media addiction

Internet and social media addiction, including phenomena like Internet addiction disorder (IAD), have become significant concerns in the contemporary digital era, affecting Muslim communities as well. While IAD is not formally recognised as a clinical disorder, challenges such as Facebook addiction and other social media dependencies are observed among Muslims. Research suggests the addictive nature of Facebook, with "Facebook addiction" describing individuals who excessively and compulsively use the platform as a means of mood alteration, leading to negative personal outcomes (Kuss & Griffiths, 2011; Andreassen & Pallesen, 2014; Chakraborty, 2017; Ryan et al., 2014). Individuals with Facebook addiction may experience a loss of control while persistently engaging in excessive Facebook use, despite adverse impacts on their lives. Individuals with IAD may exhibit warning signs and experience relapses, facing health and social consequences akin to those addicted to substances, gambling, and other compulsive behaviours. Those suffering from IAD often perceive the virtual environment as more appealing than everyday reality (Chebbi et al., 2000), leading to various physical and psychosocial consequences affecting school, family, work, marriage, and relationships. Risk factors for Internet addiction among university students include male gender, skipping breakfast, mental health issues, deficient social support, and neurotic personality characteristics (Tsai et al., 2009). Facebook addiction may manifest as preoccupation with the platform, loss of control, denial of excessive use, disrupted sleep patterns, strained relationships, compulsive behaviour, and persistent use despite negative impacts (Mehdizadeh, 2010; Andreassen et al., 2012). Personality traits such as extraversion, narcissism, high levels of neuroticism, and lower self-esteem are linked to Facebook addiction (Mehdizadeh, 2010; Andreassen et al., 2012), along with social deficits and a relationship between anxiety, depression, and compulsive Facebook use (Koc & Gulyagci, 2013; Muench et al., 2015).

Cybersex addiction

Cybersex addiction is recognised as a significant social issue and emerges when sexual behaviours spiral out of control, leading individuals to engage in obsessive sexual behaviour despite negative consequences (Rassool, 2011). Online sexual behaviours are categorised into cyber sexual consumption and cyber sexual interaction, with the former involving activities like downloading sexual content and the latter encompassing real-time or delayed interactions (Griffiths, 2012a). Cybersex addiction intersects Internet addiction and sex addiction, with some individuals using online sexual behaviour as a complement to offline sexuality while others use it as a substitute (Griffiths, 2012b). Schneider's study (2000) highlighted significant negative consequences of cybersex addiction on relationships, including separation and divorce, impacting 22.3% of respondents. Children were also affected by exposure to cyber-pornography, parental conflicts, and lack of attention due to a parent's computer involvement, emphasizing the profound impact of cybersex addiction on families.

Pornography addiction is recognised as a social issue associated with sex addiction, impacting individuals regardless of their faith or marital status. A survey by Muslim Link (2010) revealed that pornography addiction affects married men actively engaged in their faith as much as unmarried college students, with some *Imams* addressing the issue in marriage counselling sessions. Concerns raised by wives about the increasing prevalence of pornography among Muslim men prompt questions about its purpose as an outlet (Abdullah, 2007). The reasons behind pornography addiction among Muslim men remain uncertain, but there is a suggestion that it stems from a lack of proper realisation of Islāmic principles, hindering adherence to lawful practices and avoidance of harm to themselves, their families, and the community (Abdullah, 2007).

HIV/AIDS and addicted Muslims

The transmission of HIV among injecting drug users (IDUs) primarily occurs through the sharing of contaminated injection paraphernalia like needles and syringes, increasing the risk of acquiring HIV and other blood-borne infections. Alcohol and substance use disorders contribute to HIV transmission through risky sexual behaviours, further complicating the spread of the virus. People living with HIV are reported to experience more severe outcomes and increased comorbidities from COVID-19 compared to those without HIV. However, existing inequalities hinder their access to COVID-19 vaccines and essential HIV services. The impact of COVID-19 lockdowns has disrupted HIV testing, leading to significant declines in diagnoses, referrals to care services, and treatment initiations (UNAIDS, 2020). People with HIV may have higher rates of certain underlying health conditions, and older age combined with these conditions could increase the likelihood of severe illness with COVID-19. This heightened risk is particularly notable for individuals with advanced HIV, including those with an AIDS diagnosis, or those with HIV who are not on HIV treatment (Centers for Disease Control and Prevention, 2023).

The taboo nature of HIV and sexually transmitted diseases within Muslim communities stems from Islāmic beliefs prohibiting alcohol and drug use and premarital and extramarital sex. Despite the traditional perception of Muslim countries being shielded from HIV/AIDS due to religious and cultural norms, there is a growing threat globally. This shift is attributed to changing lifestyles influenced by acculturation, engaging in unprotected sexual activities, same-gender relationships, sex work, and the sharing of injection equipment. The emergence of these behaviours poses challenges to previously established norms, contributing to the rising risk of HIV/AIDS in Muslim communities worldwide.

References

Abdullah, A. L. (2007). *The secret lives of Muslim husbands.* https://islamonline.net/en/the-secret-lives-of-muslim-husbands/, (accessed 13 January 2024).

Abdul-Rahman, Z. (2023). *How to overcome addiction through faith: Ibn-Qayyim's rehabilitation programme.* Irving, TX: Yaqeen Institute.

Adiran, M. (2003). How can sociological theory help our understanding of addictions? *Substance Use & Misuse,* 38(10), 1385–1423.

Agrawal, A., & Lynskey, M. T. (2008). Are there genetic influences on addiction: evidence from family, adoption and twin studies. *Addiction,* 103(7), 1069–1081. https://doi.org/10.1111/j.1360-0443.2008.02213.x

American Psychiatric Association. (2013). *Diagnostic and statistical manual of mental disorders* (5th ed.) (DSM-V). Washington DC: American Psychiatric Association.

American Psychological Association. (2024). APA dictionary of psychology. *Addictions.* https://dictionary.apa.org/addiction?_gl=1*1*1*19hit3z*_ga* MjAxMTUzNTM5Ny4xNjc0MDM1*1OTU5*_ga_SZXLGDJGNB* MTcwNDk2MTQ4NC4xNi4wLjE3MDQ5NjE0ODDQuMC4wLjA, (accessed 10 January 2024).

American Society of Addiction Medicine. (2011). *Public policy statement: Definition of addiction.* https://www.asam.org/docs/default-source/ public-policy-statements/1definition_of_addiction_long_4-11.pdf? sfvrsn=a8f64512_4, (accessed 11 January 2024).

Andreassen, C. S., & Pallesen, S. (2014). Social network site addiction – an overview. *Current Pharmaceutical Design*, 20(25), 4053–4061. https://doi.org/10.2174/13816128113199990616

Andreassen, C. S., Torsheim, T., Brunborg, G. S., & Pallesen, S. (2012). Development of a Facebook addiction scale. *Psychological Reports*, 110(2), 501–517. https://doi.org/10.2466/02.09.18.PR0.110.2.501-517

Badri, M. (2009). The AIDS crisis: An Islāmic perspective, in Farid Esack & Sarah Chiddy (Eds.), *Islam and AIDS: Between scorn, pity and justice*. Oxford: Oneworld, pp. 28–42.

Bolton, D. (2023). A revitalized biopsychosocial model: Core theory, research paradigms, and clinical implications. *Psychological Medicine*, 53(16), 7504–7511. https://doi.org/10.1017/S0033291723002660

Centers for Disease Control and Prevention. (2023). Division of HIV Prevention, National Center for HIV, Viral Hepatitis, STD, and TB Prevention, Centers for Disease Control and Prevention. *HIV and COVID-19 basics*. https://www.cdc.gov/hiv/basics/covid-19.html, (accessed 13 January 2024).

Chakraborty, A. (2017). Facebook addiction: An emerging problem. *American Journal of Psychiatry Residents' Journal*, 11(12), 7–9. https://doi.org/10.1176/appi.ajp-rj.2016.111203

Chebbi, P., Koong, K. S., & Rottman, R. (2000). Some observations on internet addiction disorder research. *Journal of Information Systems Education*, 11(3–4), 97–99.

Drummond, D. C., Tiffany, S. T., Glautier, S., & Remington, B. (1995). Cue exposure in understanding and treating addictive behaviours, in D. C. Drummond, S. T. Tiffany, S. Glautier, & B. Remington (Eds.), *Addictive behaviour: Cue exposure theory and practice*. Oxford: John Wiley & Sons, pp. 1–17.

Engs, R. C. (1987). *Alcohol and other drugs: Self responsibility*. Bloomington, IN: Tichenor Publishing Company.

Engel, G. L. (1977). The need for a new medical model: A challenge for biomedicine. *Science*, 196(4286), 129–136.

Foster, S. L., & Weinshenker, D. (2019).Chapter 15 – The role of norepinephrine in drug addiction: Past, present, and future, in Mary Torregrossa (Ed.), *Neural mechanisms of addiction*. Cambridge, Massachusetts: Academic Press, pp. 221–236. https://doi.org/10.1016/B978-0-12-812202-0.00015-4

Ghaferi, H., Al, Bond, & Matheson, C. (2016). Does the biopsychosocial-spiritual model of addiction apply in an Islāmic context? A qualitative study of Jordanian addicts in treatment. *Drug and Alcohol Dependence*, 172, 14–20. https://doi.org/10.1016/j.drugalcdep.2016.11.019

Griffiths, M. D. (2012a). To what extent can cybersex be addictive? http://drmarkgriffiths.wordpress.com/2012/01/04/to-what-extent-can-cybersex-be-addictive/, (accessed 13 January 2024).

Griffiths M. D. (2012b). Internet sex addiction: A review of empirical research. *Addiction Research and Theory*, 20(2), 111–124.

Gupta, R., & Derevensky, J. L. (1998). Adolescent gambling behavior: A prevalence study and examination of the correlates associated with problem gambling. *Journal of Gambling Studies*, 14(4), 319–345. https://doi.org/10.1023/a:1023068925328

Hamond, A., & Rassool, G. Hussein. (2006). Spiritual and cultural needs: Integration in dual diagnosis care, in G. Hussein Rassool (Ed.), *Dual diagnosis nursing*. Oxford: Blackwell Publishing.

Ibn al-Qayyim. (2010). *Rawḍat al-muḥibbīn*, ed. Muḥammad ʿAzīz Shams. Jeddah: Dār ʿAlam al-Fawāʾid.

Ibn Majah. *Sunan Ibn Majah 3375*. In-book reference: Book 30, Hadith 5. English translation: Vol. 4, Book 30, Hadith 3375. Hasan (Darussalam). https://sunnah.com/ibnmajah:3375

Koc, M., & Gulyagci, S. (2013). Facebook addiction among Turkish college students: the role of psychological health, demographic, and usage characteristics. *Cyberpsychology, Behavior and Social Networking*, 16(4), 279–284. https://doi.org/10.1089/cyber.2012.0249

Kuss, D. J., & Griffiths, M. D. (2011). Online social networking and addiction--A review of the psychological literature. *International Journal of Environmental Research and Public Health*, 8(9), 3528–3552. https://doi.org/10.3390/ijerph8093528

Leeds, J., & Morgenstern, M. J. (1996). Psychoanalytic theories of substance abuse, in F. Rotgers, D. S. Keller and J. Morgenstern (Eds.), *Treating substance abuse: Theory and Technique*. New York: Guildford Press.

Mehdizadeh, S. (2010). Self-presentation 2.0: Narcissism and self-esteem on Facebook. *Cyberpsychology, Behavior, and Social Networking*, 13(4), 357–364. https://doi.org/10.1089/cyber.2009.0257

Merikangas, K. R., Stevens, D. E., Fenton, B., Stolar, M., O'Malley, S., Woods, S. W. & Risch, N. (1998) Co-morbidity and familial aggregation of alcoholism and anxiety disorders. *Psychological Medicine*, 28 (4), 773–788.

Muench, F., Hayes, M., Kuerbis, A., & Shao, S. (2015). The independent relationship between trouble controlling Facebook use, time spent on the site and distress. *Journal of Behavioral Addictions*, 4(3), 163–169. https://doi.org/10.1556/2006.4.2015.013

Müller, C. P., & Homberg, J. R. (2015). The role of serotonin in drug use and addiction. *Behavioural Brain Research*, 277, 146–192. https://doi.org/10.1016/j.bbr.2014.04.007

Muslim Link Staff. (2010). *Suffering in the silence: Pornography addiction*. http://www.muslimlinkpaper.com/index.php/community-news/community-news/2419-suffering-in-the-silence-pornography-addiction.html, (accessed 13 January 2024).

Orford, J. (2001). *Excessive appetites: A psychological view of addictions* (2nd ed.). Oxford: John Wiley & Sons Ltd.

Oyefeso, A., Ghodse, H., Keating, A., Annan, J., Phillips, T., Pollard. M., & Nash, P. (2000): *Drug treatment needs of Black and minority ethnic residents of the London Borough of Merton*. Addictions Resource Agency for Commissioners (ARAC) Monograph Series on Ethnic Minority Issues. London: ARAC.

Petry, N. M., Blanco, C., Auriacombe, M., Borges, G., Bucholz, K., Crowley, T. J., Grant, B. F., Hasin, D. S., & O'Brien, C. (2014). An overview of and rationale for changes proposed for pathological gambling in DSM-5. *Journal of Gambling Studies*, 30(2), 493–502. https://doi.org/10.1007/s10899-013-9370-0

Potenza, M. N. (2013). Neurobiology of gambling behaviors. *Current Opinion in Neurobiology*, 23(4), 660–667. https://doi.org/10.1016/j.conb.2013.03.004

Prescott, C. A., Khoddam, R., & Arpawong, T. E. (2016). Genetic risk for substance abuse and addiction: Family and twin studies. *Encyclopedia of Life Sciences*. https://doi.org/10.1002/9780470015902.a0005230.pub2

Rash, C. J., Weinstock, J., & Van Patten, R. (2016). A review of gambling disorder and substance use disorders. *Substance Abuse and Rehabilitation*, 7, 3–13. https://doi.org/10.2147/SAR.S83460

Rassool, G. Hussein. (2011). *Understanding addiction behaviours: Theoretical & clinical practice in health and social care*. Basingstoke, Hampshire: Palgrave McMillan.

Rassool, G. Hussein. (2018). *Alcohol and drug misuse. A guide for health and social care professionals* (2nd ed.). Oxford: Routledge.

Rassool, G. Hussein. (2020). Chapter 16: Addictive behaviours: Gambling, internet, and cybersex addiction, in G. Hussein Rassool, *Health and psychology from an Islāmic perspective*, Vol. 2. UK: Islāmic Psychology Publishing (IIP). Amazon.

Rassool, G. Hussein. (2021). *Mother of all evils: Addictive behaviours from an Islāmic perspective*. London: Islāmic Psychology Publication (IIP) & Institute of Islāmic Psychology Research (RIIPR). Amazon/Kindle.

Ryan, T., Chester, A., Reece, J., & Xenos, S. (2014). The uses and abuses of Facebook: A review of Facebook addiction. *Journal of Behavioral Addictions*, 3(3), 133–148. https://doi.org/10.1556/JBA.3.2014.016

Sher, K., Walitzer, K., Wood, P. & Brent, E. (1991) Characteristics of children of alcoholics: Putative risk factors, substance use and abuse, and psychopathology. *Journal of Abnormal Psychology*, 100 (4), 427–448.

Siddiqi, M. I. (1981). *Islam forbids intoxicants and gambling*. Lahore: Kazi Publications.

Sinha, R. (2013). The clinical neurobiology of drug craving. *Current Opinion in Neurobiology*, 23(4), 649–654. https://doi.org/10.1016/j.conb.2013.05.001

Tsai, H. F., Cheng, S. H., Yeh, T. L., Shih, C. C., Chen, K. C., Yang, Y. C., & Yang, Y. K. (2009). The risk factors of Internet addiction – a survey of university freshmen. *Psychiatry Research*, 167(3), 294–299. https://doi.org/10.1016/j.psychres.2008.01.015

UNAIDS. (2020). *AIDSinfo*. Geneva: UNAIDS. https://aidsinfo.unaids.org/, (accessed 13 January 2024).

UNODC. (2018). *World drug report 2018*. Vienna: United Nations Office on Drugs and Crime.

West, R. (2006) *Theory of addiction*. Oxford: Blackwell Publishing.

Winters, K. C., & Rich, T. (1998). A twin study of adult gambling behavior. *Journal of Gambling Studies*, 14, 213–225. https://doi.org/10.1023/A:1022084924589

2 Tracing the footsteps of addictive behaviours in Islāmic history

Introduction

The historical use of psychoactive substances such as herbs, plants, alcohol, and drugs dates back thousands of years and has been documented in ancient civilisations. These substances served various purposes including medicinal, religious, cultural, and recreational uses, often acting as social lubricants (Rassool, 2018, 2025). In ancient Mesopotamia, beer held significant symbolic and practical roles, considered a divine gift, a symbol of civilisation, a dietary staple, a facilitator of social interactions, and a crucial element in religious rituals (Paulette & Fisher, 2017). Opium's historical usage in ancient Egypt is evidenced in medical papyri, indicating its recognition for therapeutic potential within ancient medical practices (Veiga, 2016). Alcoholic beverages, common across various ancient civilisations, reveal diverse cultural, social, and religious significances attached to these substances. In ancient Greece, mead and wine held cultural importance, utilised in rituals, social gatherings, hospitality, and daily meals, with an emphasis on moderate consumption (Hanson, 1995). In China, alcohol was viewed as a spiritual sustenance integral to various facets of life, while in India, beverages like *Sura* had specific social contexts (Peele & Grant, 1999). The Roman Empire experienced a transition from ceremonial to everyday drinking, contributing to increased instances of chronic drunkenness akin to modern alcoholism (Babor, 1989). Following the empire's collapse, monasteries became custodians of brewing and winemaking techniques from the ancient world (Babor, 1989). The Industrial Revolution introduced new beverages, production methods, and drinking patterns, while contemporary times witness socioeconomic, political, and psychosocial factors influencing heavy drinking trends in regions such as Asia, Africa, and Latin America.

The term "alcohol" finds its roots in the Arabic language, possibly originating from *al-kuḥl*, associated with the production of a black powder used as eyeliner, or from *al-ġawl*, meaning spirit or demon, similar to the term "spirits" in English. It was not until the 16th century that alcohol

DOI: 10.4324/9781032669212-2

specifically referred to distilled spirits. The historical use of psychoactive substances in the Islāmic world is a multifaceted subject, influenced by religious teachings, cultural practices, and evolving social norms. The evolution of their use, from religious rituals and medications to contemporary recreational and social practices, is explored (Nicholls, 2012). This chapter examines the historical development of alcohol, drugs, caffeine, and gambling in the Islāmic world, aiming to understand the changing nature of addiction in contemporary societies and Muslim communities.

Pre-Islāmic period

During the pre-Islāmic era, known as *Jahiliyah* (The period of ignorance), Arab society was characterised by constant tribal warfare and social issues such as prostitution and female infanticide. These aspects highlight the challenging social conditions prevailing during the pre-Islāmic era (Quran & Science, 2009). In pre-Islāmic Arabia, wine consumption was associated with nobility and recreation, with archaeological findings revealing residues of psychoactive substances like wine in pottery and containers, providing tangible evidence of their use. During pre-Islāmic times, Arabs regarded wine as a symbol of generosity, offering alcoholic drinks like *nabith* made from honey, dates, wheat, barley, raisins, and sorghum to guests. Various mixtures, such as ripe and unripe dates or dates with raisins (*zahw*), were also prepared (Al-'Ali, 4:666). Wine was considered a luxury, often imported from Syria, Iraq, or Persia, and was particularly costly, affordable only by the wealthy (Hawi, 265). *Khamariyat*, odes or poems dedicated to wine, were composed during this period. Even some Muslims carried wine on the raid of Badr, as mentioned by Ibn Qutayba (2019). Alcohol consumption was widespread, with pots named *Hantam, Muzaffat, Naqir,* and *Muqaiyar* used to prepare and store alcoholic drinks (Islāmimanihsan.com). During the pre-Islāmic period, alcohol shops and bars operated around the clock, providing wines and entertainment. Taverns offering wine were widespread in towns and villages, and inns serving wine were prevalent along the roads (Masarwah, 2019). These establishments not only catered to individuals seeking alcoholic beverages but also offered travellers a place to rest and recover. It is noteworthy that the owners of these taverns, often marked with special banners, were predominantly Christians and Jews (Al-'Ali, 4:667, cited in Masarwah, 2019). After battles, both victors and vanquished turned to wine, doubling the intoxication of victory or providing solace for failure, helping individuals forget the toll of war. Sa'id (2019) noted that wine served as a means to cope with the aftermath of conflict, offering consolation and aiding in the process of overcoming the impact of bloodshed and loss. However, while wine was viewed as a social lubricant, excessive drinking and public intoxication were considered disgraceful, leading to consequences such as banishment by Arab tribes (Suror 2019; Tarfa, al-'Abd, 2019). Poppy and cannabis were unknown in pre-Islāmic Arabia, with cannabis appearing in Arabic countries in the 9th century, while the use of opium during this period remains undocumented (Ismail et al., 2023; Joni et al., 2023). This era reflected diverse attitudes towards alcohol consumption, with local customs and norms regulating its use and emphasising responsibility towards alcohol use.

In pre-Islāmic Arabia, gambling took various forms and was often associated with games of chance and divination. Ibn Abbas (may Allāh be pleased with him) described one prevalent form of gambling where participants would join in gambling for a camel. Ten people would contribute to buy a camel with ten newborn camels to be handed over at the time of weaning. They would draw lots, and the loser would leave the camel for the remaining nine. This process continued until the camel was settled on one person, while the rest would forfeit a newborn camel for nothing at the time of weaning, considered as *maysir* (Bukhârî). Ibn Abbas further mentioned that in the pre-Islāmic days of ignorance (jahiliyyah), individuals would even stake their wives and wealth while gambling, and the winner would take away both the defeated person's wife and wealth (Ibn Jarir, 2/358). This highlights the prevalence and severity of gambling practices during that era.

Islāmic period: Alcohol

With the rise of Islām, alcohol consumption was prohibited due to its potential for intoxication and harm and it underwent gradual prohibition in three phases. Initially, although the harm of alcohol was acknowledged as greater than its benefits, it was not explicitly prohibited (Al-Baqarah 2:219). However, some of the Sahabas (Companions of Prophet Muhammad (ﷺ)) refrained from alcohol due to *taqwa* (God consciousness). The second phase of prohibition occurred when Surah An-Nisa (4:43) was revealed after an incident where an Imam recited the Qur'ân incorrectly following a heavy drinking session. Believers were allowed to drink as long as they were sober during prayer times. The third and final phase of prohibition, resulting in total prohibition, was revealed in Surah al-Mā'idah (5:90–91). This phase was prompted by an incident where offensive poetry was recited under the influence of alcohol, leading to a fight and serious consequences (Al-Tabari, 2000; Ali, 2014, p. 914). The ultimate prohibition was enacted after the siege of Medina in the fifth Hijri (627 CE). Types of alcoholic beverages include *khamr* (wine made from grapes or dates), *bit'* (wine from honey), and *mizr* (beer from barley).

Muslim chemists during the Abbasid caliphate, notably Jabir ibn Hayyan, al-Kandi, and al-Razi, pioneered the isolation of ethanol (alcohol) as a pure compound through distillation (Al-Hassan & Hill, 1986;

Al-Hassan, 2001). Jabir ibn Hayyan, credited with inventing the alembic still, observed the release of flammable vapour from heated wine, deeming it "of great importance to science" despite its limited practical use (Rassool, 2018, p. 22). Al-Razi (864–930) significantly contributed by describing alcohol distillation and its medical applications (Al-Hassan & Hill, 1986). During the Islāmic Renaissance period from the 9th century, alcohol was utilised as an antiseptic (Majeed, 2005). The knowledge and techniques of alcohol distillation were later transmitted to Europe in the 12th century, where European authors popularised them through translations of works by Islāmic and Persian alchemists, contributing to the dissemination and adoption of distillation techniques in medieval Europe (Al-Hassan, 2001). This exchange of knowledge played a crucial role in the dissemination and adoption of distillation techniques and alcohol-related discoveries in medieval Europe (Al-Hassan, 2001).

Islāmic period: Drug

In early Islāmic medical treatises and the literature of *Tibb al-Nabawi*, cannabis and poppy were recognised as potent medicines to be used sparingly when necessary (Hamarneh, 1972). Early Muslim scholars acknowledged both the benefits and harmful effects of drugs, advocating for the prudent use of permissible drugs for medicinal purposes while cautioning against dangerous ones (Safian, 2013). The literature on *Fiqh* frequently mentions terms like Hashish, Banj, Khat, Nabat Majhul, and Mukhaddar to discuss drugs (Safia, 2010). Despite the recognition and availability of substances like hemp (*hashisha*), henbane (*banj*), and opium (*afyun*), there is no evidence of recreational drug use during the formative period of Islam (Rosenthal, 1971; Hamarneh, 1972). Poppy was prescribed in early Islāmic medicine by Yuhanna b. Masawayh for various ailments, including pain relief, fevers, indigestion, and inducing sleep (Hamarneh, 1972). However, Ali al-Tabari cautioned that poppy extract could be lethal, emphasising the poisonous nature of extracts and opium derived from poppy (Hamarneh, 1972).

Rosenthal (1971) suggests that evidence indicates drug use in the Muslim world dating back to the 3rd century of the *Hijra* (refers to the migration of the Prophet Muhammad (ﷺ) from Mecca to Medina in the year 622 CE), based on the prohibitions of narcotics by prominent figures like al-Muzani (d. 264/878) and al-Tahawi (d. 321/933). Rosenthal indicates an escalation of the drug problem during the late 6th and early 7th centuries of the *Hijra*, particularly after the Tartars came into power. In contrast, Safian (2013) offers a different perspective, suggesting that while drug use existed among the population, it was not widespread or significant. Safian argues that early jurists may have been ignorant about the extent of drug use during their time. This presents a divergence in opinions regarding the prevalence and awareness of drug-related matters in the historical context discussed by these scholars.

Cannabis (*al-qinnab al-hindi*) was introduced into the Arab mainland mainly from India through Persia and via interaction with Greek physicians (Hamarneh, 1972). The earliest documented therapeutic application of medical cannabis dates back to the 9th century (Fakhry et al., 2021). Rosenthal (1971) suggested that cannabis was consumed orally rather than smoked, aiding digestion (*hadim al-aqwat*) and enhancing mental clarity (*ba'ithat al-fikir*). During the medieval Islāmic civilisation era, numerous Muslim scholars extensively acknowledged and documented the medicinal use of cannabis. Lozano (2001) highlighted that Arab doctors from the 8th to the 18th centuries extensively documented the pharmacological properties of cannabis, recognising its diverse medical benefits. Muslim texts indicated that cannabis was utilised for various purposes, including as a digestive, diuretic, anti-inflammatory, anti-epileptic, painkiller, anti-flatulent, appetite stimulant, anti-emetic, antipyretic, anxiolytic, antipsychotic, anti-tumour, anti-spasmodic, and for the treatment of other ailments.

Muslim jurists contributed to the utilisation of various parts of the cannabis plant for medicinal purposes. The juice, seeds, and oil from the green seeds and leaves were commonly used to aid patients (Lozano, 2001). Muslims reportedly utilised cannabis in sedative and analgesic mixtures prescribed before surgical procedures (Ahmed et al., 2014; Oncel & Erdemir, 2007; Takrouri, 2010). Ibn al-Baytar recognised the potential of cannabis, specifically hemp seed oil, in alleviating neuropathic pain, a finding validated by recent clinical investigations (Russo, 2017). The Islāmic polymath Al-Razi documented the therapeutic properties of cannabis and emphasised its role as a pain reliever for various conditions, such as dysentery and intestinal worms. Ibn Sina also utilised different parts of the hashish plant, including seeds, leaves, and the root, to address toothaches (Taha, 2010). Furthermore, a 17th-century Persian medical book titled *Makhzon-ul-Adwiya* recorded the use of boiled hashish roots as a poultice to reduce neuralgic pains (Alakbarov, 2001).

Historical records, including Russo (2007), Golshani and Mosleh (2015), Taha (2010), Haddad (2006), Frye and Smitherman (2018), and Fakhry et al. (2021), indicate the extensive historical use of cannabis for various medical purposes. These include the treatment of ear problems, depression, epilepsy, and migraine headaches. Additionally, the Persian philosopher and scientist Ibn Sina utilised cannabis to address ear infections, skin rashes, inflammation, joint diseases, ophthalmitis, oedema, and wounds. These historical accounts highlight the diverse therapeutic applications of cannabis in traditional medicine across different cultures and historical periods. The Muslim text emphasises that there is substantial scientific data and evidence supporting the historical usage of medical cannabis as a traditional remedy by Muslim scientists. These scholars were notably advanced, being several centuries ahead of our current understanding of the medicinal properties of cannabis. Regarding the historical use of drugs, Bos (1996) suggested that while instances of individuals dying from drug overdose, particularly due to the use of a drug employed to treat forgetfulness, known as either *baladhur* (marking-nut) or *habb al-fahm* (the nut of apprehension), have been recorded, these deaths were more likely a result of medical malpractice and incorrect dosage rather than deliberate drug abuse (p. 234).

Islāmic-Ottoman period: Gambling

In Islām, gambling is strictly forbidden and is considered a spiritual disease. Scholars like Ibn Hajar al-Makki define *Al-maysir* (gambling) as any form of betting, while Al-Mahalli highlights the prohibited aspect involving the possibility of gaining luck or facing loss. The Qur'ân explicitly addresses gambling in several verses. Qur'ân 2:219 acknowledges some benefits in alcoholic drinking and gambling but emphasises their outweighing harm and sin. Al-Mā'idah 5:90 categorises intoxicants and gambling as "an abomination of Satan's handiwork," urging believers to strictly avoid them for success. These verses clearly articulate Islām's stance on gambling, deeming it undesirable due to its potential harm and association with Satan's influence. In the Ottoman Empire, gambling was officially banned, reflecting Islāmic principles, although some forms persisted in certain communities despite enforcement variations.

Islāmic period: Caffeine

Caffeine, the world's favourite psychoactive substance, has a rich history with coffee. Initially known to Arab travellers in the 6th century, coffee, originally referred to as *qahwa*, spread from Ethiopia through Yemeni traders. Used for medicinal and religious purposes, coffee reached major Islāmic cities via the annual pilgrimage. It was utilised medicinally and for religious purposes, particularly by the dervishes to stay awake during long religious practices and rituals (Ghodse, 2010). The earliest substantiated evidence of either coffee drinking or knowledge of the coffee tree is from the 15th century, in the Sufi monasteries of Yemen (Weinberg & Bealer (2001). Al-Razi highlighted its medicinal properties, and Ibn Sina explained its benefits for digestion (Mokha Bunn). Coffee houses, known as "Kaveh Kanes," emerged in Mecca, becoming intellectual hubs (Dewitt, 2021). In the major Islāmic cities, including Cairo and Istanbul, the Islāmic scholars and religious authorities discussed about the effects of coffee which they remarked as being similar to alcohol rituals. However, controversy arose with Islāmic scholars remarking on coffee's effects, likening them to alcohol rituals and "even worse than the wine room" (McHugo, 2013). Some Sufi sects used coffee at funerals to stay awake during prayers (Blotnick, 2013).

Pre-Ottoman and Ottoman period: Alcohol, drug, caffeine, and gambling

The Ottoman Empire, successor of Sunni orthodoxy, strictly adhered to the Qur'ânic prohibition of alcohol. Throughout Ottoman history, records are full of instances of persecutions against those who dared to consume forbidden beverages. The Ottoman perspective reflected a commitment to upholding Islāmic principles, resulting in a rigorous enforcement of anti-alcohol measures, even as the empire navigated a diverse and cosmopolitan cultural landscape (Rassool, 2022). During the rule of Sultan Süleyman the Magnificent in the Ottoman Empire, alcohol was prohibited. Sultan Süleyman extended the ban on wine-drinking to Muslims and implemented measures such as dismissing palace dancers and musicians, replacing silver plates with earthenware, and ordering the burning of musical instruments set with gold and precious stones. To enforce this prohibition, he enacted laws stipulating severe punishment, including pouring melted lead down the throats of those found drunk. However, this policy was reversed during the reign of Selim II (1566–1574). It is reported that "While still heir to the throne, his friend Celal Bey warned him that his love of pleasure was eroding his authority and esteem. Draining his glass of wine, Selim replied, 'I live for today, and think not of tomorrow.'" (Işın, 2022). Sultan Bayezid I initially drank wine until experiencing shame and repentance.

Subsequent Ottoman rulers, including Sultan Ahmed I, reinstated and enforced bans on alcohol consumption. In 1613, Sultan Ahmed I ordered the demolition of drinking houses in Istanbul and the destruction of liquor kegs. Sultan Murad IV took extreme measures, personally patrolling the streets in disguise, executing drunkards on the spot. Following this era, Ottoman sultans refrained from excessive drinking, and only water, sherbet, and coffee were approved beverages for Muslims both in the palace and throughout the empire (Işın, 2022). During Abdul Hamid II's reign (1842–1918) as the 34th Sultan of the Ottoman Empire, he faced political and economic pressures from European colonial powers, leading to increased reliance on the West. Despite his adherence to traditional Islāmic spirituality, the Ottoman Empire saw the establishment of the first *rakı* (a Turkish alcoholic drink) and beer factories. The Bomonti Brothers opened the first beer factory in Istanbul, and the Olympus Brewery was established in Thessaloniki during this period (www.britishdeepstate.com, 2017).

Coffee houses flourished in the empire, serving as hubs for social inter-action and intellectual discourse, making coffee a symbol of Ottoman cul-ture and hospitality. The first recorded coffee crackdown occurred in Mecca in 1511, when Khaʻir Beg al-Miʻmar, a prominent secular official in a pre-Ottoman regime, caught men drinking coffee outside of a mosque and thought they looked suspicious. The details of the crackdown are dis-puted, but he used religious justifications to order an end to all coffee sales and consumption (Hay, 2018). In 1511, the orthodox *Imams* of Makkah banned coffee because the Islāmic tradition condemns any type of poison-ing. But in itself, the prohibition was due to the rumours that reached the emir Khair Bey from the "Kaveh Kanes" (Dewitt, 2021). Sultan Selim I lifted the ban in 1524, leading to the growth of coffee houses. Later coffee crackdowns occurred in Makkah (again), Cairo (multiple times), and Istanbul and other Ottoman areas (Hay, 2018). A cluster of coffee houses grew up in the vast Ottoman Turkish Empire in 1554. Coffee houses became a meeting for recreation and a focus for intellectual life and could be seen as an implicit rival to the mosque as a meeting place (McHugo, 2013). Sultan Murad IV reinstated the ban in 1623 and set up a system of reasonable penalties. The punishment for a first offence was a beating. Anyone caught with coffee a second time was sewn into a leather bag and thrown into the waters of the Bosphorus (Blotnick, 2013). In the early 17th century, coffee faced opposition and subsequent rebellions in Egypt, particularly in the city of Cairo. The resistance to coffee was likely rooted in cultural and religious conservatism, with some viewing it as a disruptive force in society. By the year 1630, the city of Cairo saw the proliferation of coffee houses, reaching a significant number. These coffee houses became popular social spaces, fostering interaction, discussion, and intellectual exchange among diverse groups of people. Religious scholars, often influ-ential in matters of societal norms and practices, played a crucial role in shaping the perception of coffee. Over time, these scholars revisited the issue and engaged in discussions about the permissibility of consuming coffee. As a result of their deliberations, a consensus emerged among reli-gious authorities that deemed coffee permissible, indicating that it did not violate Islāmic principles. It is worth noting that during the colonial period in Brazil, it is the Muslim slaves from West Africa possessed more knowledge about coffee than their Portuguese masters (José Reis, 1995). This phenomenon is attributed to the cultural background and long his-tory of coffee consumption in West African regions, such as Ethiopia, where coffee originated, had a long history of coffee consumption. By the end of the 18th century, coffee had undergone a remarkable transforma-tion from a local beverage to one of the world's most profitable export commodities.

Gambling was a significant social issue during the Second Constitutional Period in Istanbul, which was part of the Ottoman Empire.

Increased actions such gambling and debauchery, during this period, indicate the existence of social and moral decay (Şahin, 2020). The social and moral fabric of society was shaken, leading to damage in the family structure, and even the reputation of the state, particularly as gambling became widespread among civil servants (Şahin, 2020). Despite the Ottoman government's efforts to address the issue of gambling during the Second Constitutional Period, preventive measures, legal regulations, and police interventions proved ineffective in curbing the prevalence of gambling (Şahin, 2020).

Contemporary era

In the contemporary Islāmic world, attitudes towards alcohol, drug use, coffee consumption, and gambling exhibit considerable diversity. While some nations strictly prohibit alcohol and drugs, others permit consumption with varying degrees of restriction, reflecting diverse interpretations of religious teachings and cultural norms. Coffee remains a cherished beverage in Islāmic societies, valued for its taste and cultural significance, although concerns regarding excessive caffeine consumption persist. Gambling is generally outlawed in most Muslim-majority countries, although some have legalised specific forms for tourism purposes, prompting ongoing discussions about permissibility and potential harm.

The issue of addiction within Muslim communities is not extensively studied, and there is limited available data on illicit drug use, tobacco, and gambling among Muslims. Existing research, particularly on religious minorities in Western countries, has mainly focused on high school students (Abu-Ras et al., 2010; Ahmed et al., 2014; Arfken & Ahmed, 2016). Determining the prevalence of alcohol and drug use/abuse among Muslims is challenging due to the stigma associated with self-reporting such behaviours. However, addiction remains a significant social and public health concern in both Muslim-majority countries and among Muslim minorities in Western nations. Addressing these challenges requires an understanding of cultural, religious, and social factors influencing attitudes and behaviours towards substance use and gambling within Muslim communities.

Alcohol

Alcohol consumption in the Muslim world presents a complex picture that challenges the assumption of universal abstinence dictated by Islāmic faith. Recent studies highlight a notable increase in alcohol consumption in Muslim-majority countries (ANSAMed, 2011). The Economist (2012) reported rising alcohol use in several nations, with Lebanon and Turkey showing the highest consumption rates. However, alcohol consumption rates in countries like Egypt, Tunisia, Morocco, and the UAE are often influenced by tourism and the presence of expatriates. In places where alcohol is legal, such as Lebanon and Turkey, bars and nightlife establishments thrive. Although the prevalence of alcohol consumption in Iran is lower than in developed countries, there is a considerable variation in the alcohol consumption at the provincial level as well as in different gender groups (Rezaei et al., 2022). This has prompting the establishment of alcohol rehabilitation centres that recognise addiction as an illness (Samimi, 2013). International surveys have further revealed instances of alcohol indulgence among Muslim students in Lebanon (Ghandour et al., 2007).

The World Health Organization's (WHO) Eastern Mediterranean Region and Muslim-majority countries like Niger, Indonesia, and Azerbaijan exhibit low per capita alcohol consumption, with abstinence rates of ≥80% being the highest in Muslim-majority countries in North Africa and the Eastern Mediterranean (WHO, 2018, p. 41). In the United Kingdom, South Asians, particularly those from Pakistani and Bangladeshi backgrounds, show high abstinence rates, but among drinkers, especially Pakistani and Muslim men, heavy drinking is common (Hurcombe et al., 2010). Turkish and Moroccan immigrants in the Netherlands report less alcohol use compared to the Dutch population (Monshouwer et al., 2007; Hosper et al., 2007). In the United States, Muslim participants consider episodic excessive drinking normative for their age group but believe it should cease upon marriage and parenthood (Arfken et al., 2012). Studies in Israel and Canada reveal hidden alcohol consumption among young Muslim men (Eseed & Khoury-Kassabri, 2018) and Somali Canadians, respectively (Agic et al., 2011).

Drugs and tobacco

The misuse of opiates, including opium and heroin, is widespread in South-West Asian and South Asian countries, notably Iran, Pakistan, and Afghanistan. In Pakistan, around 8.9 million people are affected, primarily consuming cannabis and opioids (Hayat et al., 2018). High rates of opioid use are documented in up to 12 Arab countries, with Bahrain and Kuwait reporting particularly elevated rates (Wilby & Wilbur, 2017). The Middle East and North Africa (MENA) region, identified by the Joint United Nations Programme on HIV/AIDS (UNAIDS) as experiencing a deteriorating HIV epidemic, are especially vulnerable due to non-sterile opioid injection practices (UNAIDS, 2021). In Iran, tramadol misuse is reported, and in Kazakhstan, approximately 1% of the adult population is estimated to be injecting drugs. Traditional opium alkaloids use, like morphine and codeine, is noted in Kazakhstan's cultural history, especially in the drink *koknar* (Olcott & Udalova, 2000, p. 9). Nigeria, Egypt, and Tunisia also face challenges related to opioid misuse, including tramadol, codeine, morphine, and buprenorphine. Adolescents in Algeria and Morocco reportedly use heroin, indicating the widespread issue of opiate misuse in diverse regions (UNDOC, 2021a).

Cannabis cultivation is widespread in various countries with both Muslim-majority and minority populations, including Morocco, Egypt, Nigeria, Albania, Turkey, Afghanistan, Lebanon, Pakistan, Kyrgyzstan, Kazakhstan, Azerbaijan, India, and Indonesia (UNDOC, 2021a). Morocco remains a significant source country for globally intercepted cannabis resin, along with Afghanistan, Pakistan, and Lebanon (UNDOC, 2021a). In Muslim-majority countries, the production and use of substances like amphetamine-type stimulants and novel psychoactive substances have been reported (UNDOC, 2015). Afghanistan, Iraq, and the Middle East, particularly Saudi Arabia, are involved in the production and trafficking of methamphetamine, with Captagon being a prevalent drug (UNDOC, 2021b, p. 21). The final destinations of "Captagon are mostly within the sub-region, notably Saudi Arabia and various Gulf countries (including Qatar and the UAE)" (UNDOC, 2021b, p. 72). Saudi Arabia primarily consumes "Captagon," known as *Abu Hilalain*, alongside khat and hashish. Iraq is concerned about Captagon, crystalline methamphetamine, and tramadol. Methamphetamine is emerging in Afghanistan, often used with opiates. The Islamic Republic of Iran reports common methamphetamine use among people with opioid use disorders. Low levels of ecstasy use are observed in various countries, including Kazakhstan, Afghanistan, and Nigeria. Crystalline methamphetamine use is reported in Indonesia, and Bangladesh faces widespread use of amphetamine-type stimulants, especially in urban areas.

Khat, a stimulant, is widely used in East Africa, Yemen, and Southern Saudi Arabia, with an estimated 10 million users worldwide. In Somalia and Yemen, up to 80% of adults reportedly use khat. Its usage has spread to immigrant African communities in the United Kingdom, Europe, the United States, Canada, and Australia. Khat is banned in several countries, including Saudi Arabia, Egypt, Morocco, Sudan, Kuwait, Canada, the United States, and various European countries. In Australia, importation is controlled by licensing, and seizures of khat and its derivatives have occurred in 51 countries globally. Studies indicate high prevalence, with 72% of males and 33% of females in Yemen reporting khat use (Al-Mugahed, 2008). In Somali communities in Australia, khat is culturally accepted and integrated into religious activities (Douglas and Abdi Hersi, 2010; Omar et al., 2015). In the United Kingdom, consumption is primarily limited to diaspora communities, including Ethiopians, Somalis, Yemenis, and some Kenyans (Anderson & Carrier, 2011).

Smoking was introduced to Muslim countries by Europeans around 1000 AH, following its spread in the West (Shafey et al., 2003). In Europe, smoking prevalence remains high among Muslims, especially men (Ghouri et al., 2006). Jordan, Indonesia, Lebanon, Bosnia and Herzegovina, and Bahrain rank high in cigarette consumption, with Yemen and Djibouti exhibiting extremely high male smoking rates. Large Arab countries like Lebanon, Jordan, Egypt, Tunisia, Syria, and Iraq also show very high rates of smoking among adult males (Ghouri et al., 2006). Estimates suggest that 60% of lung cancer patients in the UAE are smokers (Centre for Arab Genomic Studies, 2012). Turkey and Nigeria also report significant smoking rates, while in Malaysia, urban areas exhibit higher smoking prevalence than rural ones (Taha, 1982). In England, smoking rates vary among Muslims, with 18.4% of Muslim men and 3.9% of Muslim women being current smokers. A community survey among Muslims in New York City and surrounding areas reveals the complexity of tobacco use, including cigarette and water-pipe smoking (shisha or hookah), as well as chewing tobacco (*pân/gutka*) (Sayeed, 2011). Moreover, the prevalence of smoking cigarettes and waterpipes appears to be alarmingly high among university students in Arab countries (Nasser et al., 2020).

Waterpipe tobacco smoking (WTS), commonly known as hookah or shisha smoking, is increasing globally, particularly in the Middle East region, with hookah cafés becoming popular in European countries (Nakkash et al., 2011). Studies indicate high rates of hookah smoking among male high school students in Baghdad (Al-Delaimy & Al-Ani, 2021), as well as significant prevalence among medical and dental students in Karachi, Pakistan (cited in Khan, 2020). Interestingly, hookah smoking is gaining acceptance among young females in conservative Arab societies, with varying rates reported across different countries. For instance, Tunisia shows a low prevalence of 0.2%, while university students in Egypt exhibit a high prevalence of 37.8% (Dar-Odeh & Abu-Hammad, 2011). Research in Saudi Arabia indicates a high prevalence of shisha use among university students (Muzammil et al., 2019), and comparisons across Palestine, Jordan, and Turkey reveal differing percentages of current shisha smokers, with Palestinians having the highest prevalence at 36.11% (Hawash et al., 2019).

Conclusion

The journey of addictive behaviours in Islāmic history spans various substances such as alcohol, drugs, caffeine, and gambling. In pre-Islāmic times, alcohol served as a coping mechanism amid tribal conflicts, while psychoactive substances like opium and cannabis were introduced for medicinal purposes, reflecting cultural and religious intersections. The first Islāmic state in Madina banned alcohol and gambling based on Qur'ânic injunctions and *hadīth*. During the Islāmic Renaissance, there was an acknowledgement of the medicinal benefits of substances like cannabis, while alcohol and gambling were generally discouraged. The Ottoman Empire experienced periods of prohibition under different rulers, reflecting the complex relationship between Islāmic values and substance use. In the modern era, attitudes towards addictive behaviours vary across Muslim-majority countries, with alcohol and drug use generally illegal but with variations in the types and extent of drugs. Coffee remains a staple in many Islāmic societies, while gambling is illegal in most Muslim-majority countries. Opiate use poses significant public health challenges, particularly in countries like Pakistan and Iran, while cannabis cultivation contributes to global drug trade issues. Understanding the complexity of addictive behaviours in Islāmic history underlines the importance of considering cultural, historical, and religious contexts when addressing contemporary challenges associated with substance use and addiction in Muslim communities.

References

Abu-Ras, W., Ahmed, S., & Arfken, C. L. (2010). Alcohol use among U.S. Muslim college students: Risk and protective factors. *Journal of Ethnicity in Substance Abuse*, 9, 216–220.

Agic, B., Mann, R. E., & Kobus-Matthews, M. (2011). Alcohol use in seven ethnic communities in Ontario: A qualitative investigation. *Drugs: Education, Prevention and Policy*, 18(2), 116–123.

Ahmed, S., Abu-Ras, W., & Arfken, C. L. (2014). Prevalence of risk behaviors among U.S. Muslim college students. *Journal of Muslim Mental Health*, 8(1), 5.

Al-'Ali, al-Mufassal fi Tarikh al-'Arab qabla al-Islām. Cited in Masarwah, N. (2019). *The development of tropes in Arabic wine poetry up to the 12th century AD*. Newcastle upon Tyne: Cambridge Scholars Publishing.

Alakbarov, F. U. (2001). Medicinal properties of cannabis according to medieval manuscripts of Azerbaijan. *Journal of Cannabis Therapeutics*, 1(2), 3–14. https://doi.org/10.1300/J175v01n02_02

Al-Delaimy, A. K., & Al-Ani, W. A. T. (2021). Prevalence of hookah smoking and associated factors among male high school students in Iraq. *BMC Public Health*, 21, 1317. https://doi.org/10.1186/s12889-021-11386-4

Al-Hassan, A. Y. (2001). *The different aspects of Islāmic culture, science and technology in Islām*, Vol. 4, Part II. Cambridge University Press, Cambridge: UNESCO.

Al-Hassan, A. Y., & Hill, D. (1986). *Islāmic technology, an illustrated history*. Cambridge University Press, Cambridge: UNESCO.

Ali, M. (2014). Perspectives on drug addiction in Islāmic history and theology. *Religions*, 5(3), 912–928. https://doi.org/10.3390/rel5030912

Al-Mahalli in *Al-Minhaj bi Hâsyiyah al-Qalyubi*. Cited in Gambling in the Islāmic view – Definition – Law – Prohibition. https://azIslām.com/gambling-in-the-Islāmic-view-definition-law-prohibition, (accessed 14 January 2024).

Al-Mugahed, L. (2008). Khat chewing in Yemen: Turning over a new leaf. *Bulletin World Health Organization*, 86(10), 741–742.

Al-Tabari. (2000). Muhammad Ibn Jarir al-Tabari. *Jami' al-Bayan fi Ta'wil al-Qur'an*. Beirut: Mu'assassat al-Risala.

Anderson, D. M., & Carrier, N. C. M. (2011). *Khat: Social harms and legislation: A literature review*. Occasional Paper. London: Home Office.

ANSAMed. (2011). *Islām: Survey, alcohol use in mideast-Africa +25% in 5 years*. http://www.webcitation.org/query?url=http://www.ansamed. info/en/news/ME.XEF93985.html&date=2011-02-25, (accessed 15 September 2024).

Arfken, C. L., & Ahmed, S. (2016). Ten years of substance use research in Muslim populations: Where do we go from here? *Journal of Muslim Mental Health*, 10(1)13–24.

Arfken, C. L., Owens, D., & Said, M. (2012). Binge drinking among Arab/Chaldeans: An exploratory study. *Journal of Ethnicity in Substance Abuse*, 11(4), 277–293. https://doi.org/10.1080/15332640.2012.735163

Babor, T. (1989) *Alcohol – customs and rituals*. London: Burke Publishing Company Limited.

Blotnick, E. (2013). *5 historical attempts to ban coffee*. https://www.mentalfloss.com/article/12662/5-historical-attempts-ban-coffee, (accessed 14 January 2024).

Bos, G. (1996). 'Baladhur' (marking nut): A medieval drug for strengthening memory. *Bulletin of the School of Oriental and African Studies*, 59(2), 229–236.

Bukhârî. *Al-Adab Al-Mufrad*. Cited in Salahi, A. (2004). Prohibition of all types of gambling. https://www.arabnews.com/node/249764, (accessed 14 January 2024).

Centre for Arab Genomic Studies. (2012). 60% of lung cancer patients in UAE are smokers. https://gulfnews.com/uae/health/60-of-lung-cancer-patients-in-uae-are-smokers--expert-1.975887, (accessed 15 January 2024).

Dar-Odeh, N. S., & Abu-Hammad, O. A. (2011). The changing trends in tobacco smoking for young Arab women; narghile, an old habit with a liberal attitude. *Harm Reduction Journal*, 8, 24. https://doi.org/10.1186/1477-7517-8-24

Dewitt, D. (2021). *Who invented coffee? – Coffee history explained*. https://thecozycoffee.com/history-of-coffee/, (accessed 14 January 2024).

Douglas, H., & Abdi Hersi, A. (2010). Khat and Islāmic legal perspectives: Issues for consideration. *The Journal of Legal Pluralism and Unofficial Law*, 42(62), 95–114.

Eseed, R., & Khoury-Kassabri, M. (2018). Alcohol use among Arab Muslim adolescents: A mediation-moderation model of family, peer, and community factors. *The American Journal of Orthopsychiatry*. 88(1), 88–98.

Fakhry, B., Abdulrahim, M., & Chahine, M. N. (2021). Medical cannabis in Lebanon: History & therapeutic, ethical, and social challenges. A Narrative Review. *Archives of Clinical and Biomedical Research*, 5(2), 137–157.

Frye, P. C., & Smitherman, D. (2018). *The medical marijuana guide*. Lanham, Maryland: Rowman & Littlefield.

Georgeon, F. (2002). *Ottomans and drinkers: The consumption of wine and alcohol in Istanbul in the nineteenth century*. https://www.researchgate.net/publication/292235981_Ottomans_and_drinkers_The_consumption_of_alcohol_in_istanbul_in_the_nineteenth_century, (accessed 15 January 2024).

Ghandour, L. Maalouf, W., & Karam, E. (2007). *Alcohol abuse and dependence among college students in Lebanon: Exploring the role of religiosity in different religious faiths*. National Institute of Drug Abuse. https://www.drugabuse.gov/international/abstracts/alcohol-abuse-dependence-among-college-students-in-lebanon-exploring-role-religiosity-in-different, (accessed 15 January 2024).

Ghodse, H. (2010). *Ghodse's drugs and addictive behaviour: A guide to treatment*. Cambridge: Cambridge University Press.

Ghouri, N., Atcha, M., and Sheikh, A. (2006). Influence of Islām on smoking among Muslims. *BMJ*, 2006(332), 291. https://doi.org/10.1136/bmj.332.7536.291

Golshani, S. A., & Mosleh, G. (2015). Drugs and pharmacology in the Islāmic middle era. *Pharmaceutical Historian*, 45(3), 64–69.

Haddad, F. S. (2006). Some spotlights over the past 40 years. *The Middle East Journal of Anesthesiology*, 18(5), 807–824.

Hamarneh, S. (1972). Pharmacy in medieval Islām and the history of drug addiction. *Medical History*, 16(3), 226–237.

Hanson, D. J. (1995). *History of alcohol and drinking around the world*. Wesport, CT: Praeger.

Hawash, M., Mosleh, R., Hanani, A., Jarar, Y., & Hajyousef, Y. (2019). A comparison of Shisha smoking among university students in Palestine, Jordan and Turkey. *Researchsquare*. https://doi.org/10.21203/rs.2.18834/v1

Hawi, Fann al-Shi'r al-Khamri wa-Ttawuruh 'inda al-'Arab, 265. Cited in Masarwah, N. (2019). *The development of tropes in Arabic wine poetry up to the 12th century AD*. Newcastle upon Tyne: Cambridge Scholars Publishing.

Hay, M. (2018). *In Istanbul, drinking coffee in public was once punishable by death*. https://www.atlasobscura.com/articles/was-coffee-ever-illegal, (accessed 14 January 2024).

Hayat, K., Ejaz, M. & Umer, S. (2018). Birds eye view of addiction problem in Pakistan. *Global Journal of Addiction & Rehabilitation Medicine*, 6(2), 22–23.

Hosper, K., Nierkens, V., Nicolaou, M., & Stronks, K. (2007). Behavioural risk factors in two generations of non-Western migrants: Do trends converge towards the host population? *European Journal of Epidemiology*, 22(3), 163–172.

Hurcombe, R., Bayley, M, & Goodman, A. (2010). *Ethnicity and alcohol: A review of the UK literature*. New York: Joseph Rowntree Foundation.

Ibn Hajar al-Makki in *Az-Zawajir 'an Iqtirafil Kaba'ir, 2/200* Cited in Gambling in the Islāmic View – Definition – Law – Prohibition. https://azIslām.com/gambling-in-the-Islāmic-view-definition-law-prohibition, (accessed 14 January 2024).

Ibn Jarir. *Tafsir Ibn Jarir*, 2/358. Cited in Clarke, A. J. (2023). The Fiqh of Gambling, Betting and Competitions in Islām. https://thehalallife. co.uk/the-fiqh-of-gambling-betting-and-competitions-in-Islām/, (accessed 14 January 2024).

Ibn Qutayba. (2019). Adab al-Katib, 38. Cited in Masarwah, N. (2019). *The development of tropes in Arabic wine poetry up to the 12th century AD*. Newcastle upon Tyne: Cambridge Scholars Publishing, p. 15.

Işın, P. M. (2022). A forbidden pleasure – Wine drinking in Ottoman Turkey. http://www.turkish-cuisine.org/drinks-6/alcoholic-drinks-92/ wine-97.html, (accessed 15 January 2024).

Islāmimanihsan.com. Islāmic Studies Paper 1 Section A Arabia, in *The pre Islāmic period*. http://Islāmimanihsan.com/wp-content/uploads/2021/06/ Paper-1-Section-A-Arabia-In-The-Pre-Islāmic-Period.pdf, (accessed 13 January 2024).

Ismail, S. M., Joni, E. K. E., & Nordin, R. (2023). The legality of medical Cannabis from the Islāmic perspective. *Journal of Law and Society (JUUM)*, 32, 55–71. https://doi.org/10.17576/juum-2023-32-06

Joni, E. K. E., Ismail, S. M., & Nordin, R. (2023). The medicinal use of cannabis documented by Muslim scientists. *International Journal of Academic Research in Business and Social Sciences*, 13(2), 590–601.

José Reis, J. (1995). *Slave rebellion in Brazil: The Muslim uprising of 1835 in Bahia* (2nd ed.). Baltimore: The Johns Hopkins University Press, p. 96.

Khan, J. A. (2020). *The Shisha habit: A global epidemic*. Insights. *Omnia-Health*. https://insights.omnia-health.com/reports/shisha-habit-global-epidemic, (accessed 15 January 2024).

Lozano, I. (2001). The therapeutic use of Cannabis sativa (L.) in Arabic medicine. *Journal of Cannabis Therapeutics*, 1(1), 63–70. https://doi. org/10.1300/J175v01n01_05

Majeed, A. (2005). How Islām changed medicine. *BMJ*, 2005, 331. https:// doi.org/10.1136/bmj.331.7531.1486

Masarwah, N. (2019), *The development of tropes in Arabic wine poetry up to the 12th century AD*. Newcastle upon Tyne: Cambridge Scholars Publishing.

McHugo, J. (2013). *Coffee and qahwa: How a drink for Arab mystics went global*. https://www.bbc.com/news/magazine-22190802, (accessed 14 January 2024).

Mokha Bunn. *Yemen coffee history*. https://mokhabunn.ca/yemeni-coffee-history/, (accessed 14 January 2024).

Monshouwer, K., Van Dorsselaer, S., Van Os, J., Drukker, M., De Graaf, R., Ter Bogt, T., Verdurmen, J., & Vollebergh, W. (2007). Ethnic composition of schools affects episodic heavy drinking only in ethnic-minority students. *Addiction*, 102(5), 722–729.

Muzammil, Al Asmari, Al Rethaiaa, A. S., Al Mutairi, A. S., Al Rashidi, T. H., Rasheedi, H. A., & Al Rasheedi, S. A. (2019). Prevalence and perception of Shisha smoking among university students: A cross-sectional study. *Journal of International Society of Preventive & Community Dentistry*, 9(3), 275–281.

Nakkash, R. T., Khalil, J., & Afifi, R. A. (2011). The rise in narghile (shisha, hookah) waterpipe tobacco smoking: A qualitative study of perceptions of smokers and non-smokers. *BMC Public Health*, 11, 315. https://doi.org/10.1186/1471-2458-11-315

Nasser, A. M. A., Geng, Y., & Al-Wesabi, S. A. (2020). The prevalence of smoking (cigarette and waterpipe) among university students in some Arab countries: A systematic review. *Asian Pacific Journal of Cancer Prevention: APJCP*, 21(3), 583–591. https://doi.org/10.31557/APJCP.2020.21.3.583

Nicholls, J. (2012). *Review of alcohol in world history*, (review no. 1452) https://reviews.history.ac.uk/review/1452, (accessed 13 January 2024).

Olcott, M. B., & Udalova, N. (2000). *Drug trafficking on the great silk road: The security environment in central Asia.* Washington, D.C: Carnegie Endowment for International Peace.

Omar, Y. S., Jenkins, A., Altena, M. V., Tuck, H., Hynan, C., Tohow, A., Chopra, P., & Castle, D. (2015). Khat use: What is the problem and what can be done? *BioMed Research International*, 472302. https://doi.org/10.1155/2015/472302

Oncel, O., & Erdemir, A. D. (2007). A view of the development of some anaesthetic and analgesic drugs in the western world and in Turkey and some original documents. *38th International Congress for the History of Pharmacy*, 1–6.

Paulette, T., & Fisher, M. (2017). *Potent potables of the past: Beer and brewing in Mesopotamia.* https://www.researchgate.net/publication/350374205_Potent_Potables_of_the_Past_Beer_Brewing_in_Mesopotamia, (accessed 13 January 2024).

Peele, S., & Grant, M. (Eds.) (1999). *Alcohol and pleasure: A health perspective.* Philadelphia: Brunner/Mazel, p. 102.

Quran & Science. (2009). *Alcohol in Islām.* https://www.quranandscience.com/quran-science/legislative/183-alcohol-in-Islām, (accessed 13 January 2024).

Rassool, G. Hussein. (2018). *Alcohol and drug misuse. A guide for health and social care professional* (2nd ed.). Oxford: Routledge.

Rassool, G. Hussein. (2022). *Alcohol: The forbidden nectar – An Islāmic perspective.* Islāmic Psychology Publishing (IPP) &Institute of Islāmic Psychology Research (RIIPR). Amazon/Kindle.

Rassool, G. Hussein. (2025). *Alcohol and drug misuse. A guide for health and social care professional* (3rd ed.). Oxford: Routledge.

Rezaei, N., Ahmadi, N., Shams Beyranvand, M., Hasan, M., Gohari, K., Yoosefi, M., Djalalinia, S., Saeedi Moghaddam, S., Modirian, M., Pazhuheian, F., Mahdavihezaveh, A., Moradi, G., Delavari, F., Larijani, B., & Farzadfar, F. (2022). Alcohol consumption and related disorders in Iran: Results from the National Surveillance of Non-Communicable Diseases' Survey (STEPs) 2016. *PLOS Glob Public Health*, 18(11), e0000107. https://doi.org/10.1371/journal.pgph.0000107

Rosenthal. F. (1971). *The herb: Hashish versus medieval Muslim society.* Leiden: E.J. Brill.

Russo, E. B. (2007). History of cannabis and its preparations in saga, science, and sobriquet. *Chemistry and Biodiversity*, 4(8), 1614–1648. https://doi.org/10.1002/cbdv.200790144

Russo E. B. (2017). Cannabis and epilepsy: An ancient treatment returns to the fore. *Epilepsy & Behavior: E&B*, 70(Pt B), 292–297. https://doi.org/10.1016/j.yebeh.2016.09.040

Sa'id (2019), al-Khamriyyat fi al-Shi'r al-'Arabi min al-Jahiliyya ila abi Nuwwas. Cited in Masarwah, N. (2019). *The Development of Tropes in Arabic Wine Poetry up to the 12th Century AD*. Newcastle upon Tyne: Cambridge Scholars Publishing, p.15.

Safia, Y. H. M. (2010). An analysis on Islāmic rules on drugs. *International Journal of Education and Research*, 1(9), 1–16.

Safian, Y. H. (2013). An analysis on Islamic rules on drugs. *International Journal of Education and Research*, 1 (9), 1–16.

Şahin, F. K. (2020). Gambling Malady as a social problem during the second constitutional period in Istanbul. *Belleten – The Turkish Historical Society*, 84(301), 1143–1174.

Samimi, M. (2013). Iran opens first alcohol rehab center. *al-Monitor*, 25 October 2013. http://www.al-monitor.com/pulse/originals/2013/10/iran-alcohol-permit-rehab-c, (accessed 15 January 2024).

Sayeed, S. (2011). Tobacco use among Muslims in New York City and surrounding areas: Results of the Nafis Salaam community survey. *Journal of the Islāmic Medical Association of North America*, 43(1), 10–21.

Shafey, O., Dolwick, S., & Guindon, G. E. (Eds.). (2003). *Tobacco control country profiles* (2nd ed.). Atlanta, GA: America Cancer Society.

Suror (2019). Tarikh al-Hadara al-Islāmiyya fi al-Sharq min 'ahd nufoth al-Atrak ila muntasaf al-qrn al-Khamis al-Hijri, 20. Cited in Masarwah, N. (2019). *The development of tropes in Arabic wine poetry up to the 12th century AD*. Newcastle upon Tyne: Cambridge Scholars Publishing.

Taha, A. (1982). *The growing threat. Smoking and the Muslim world*. London: Ta-Ha Publishers Ltd.

Taha, J. M. (2010). Unknown contributions of the Arab and Islāmic medicine in the field of Anesthesia in the West. *Journal of the International Society for the History of Islāmic Medicine (JISHIM)*, 6–7(11–14), 1–134. https://doi.org/10.1080/03085694.2018.1400268

Takrouri, M. S. (2010). Historical essay: An Arabic surgeon, Ibn al Quff's (1232–1286) account on surgical pain relief. *Anesthesia: Essays and Researches*, 4(1), 4. https://doi.org/10.4103/0259-1162.69298

Tarfa, al-'Abd. (2019) Diwan, 31. Cited in Masarwah, N. (2019). *The development of tropes in Arabic wine poetry up to the 12th century AD*. Newcastle upon Tyne: Cambridge Scholars Publishing.

The Economist. (2012). Tequila Ummah. Alcohol in the Muslim world. *The Economist* online, Aug 17th, 2012. http://www.economist.com/blogs/graphicdetail/2012/08/daily-chart-2, (accessed 15 January 2024).

UNAIDS. (2021). End inequalities. End AIDS. Global AIDS strategy 2021–2026. https://www.unaids.org/sites/default/files/media_asset/global-AIDS-strategy-2021-2026_en.pdf, (accessed 15 January 2024).

UNDOC. (2015). *World drug report 2015*. Vienna: United Nations Office on Drugs and Crime.

UNDOC. (2021a). *The world drug report 2021. Booklet 3. Market trends: Cannabis and opioids.* Vienna: United Nations Office on Drugs and Crime.

UNDOC. (2021b). *The world drug report 2021. Booklet 4. Market trends: Cocaine amphetamine-type stimulants.* Vienna: United Nations Office on Drugs and Crime.

Veiga, P. (2016). Opium: Was it used as a recreational drug in ancient Egypt?, in Ilaria Micheli (Ed.), *Cultural and linguistic transition explored. Proceedings of the ATrA closing workshop Trieste,* May 25–26, 2016, Trieste, EUT Edizioni Università di Trieste, 2017, pp. 199–215.

Weinberg, B. A., & Bealer, B. K. (2001). *The world of caffeine: The science and culture of the world's most popular drug.* London: Routledge.

Wilby, K. J., & Wilbur, K. (2017). Cross-national analysis of estimated narcotic utilization for twelve Arabic speaking countries in the Middle East. *Saudi Pharmaceutical Journal,* 25(1), 83–87.

World Health Organization. (2018).*Global status report on alcohol and health 2018.* Geneva: WHO.

www.britishdeepstate.com (2017). *Moral decline speeds up in the Ottoman society as alcohol, gambling and adultery spread.* https://www.britishdeepstate.com/3-moral-decline-speeds-up-in-the-ottoman-society-as-alcohol-gambling-and-adultery-spread/, (accessed 15 January 2024).

3 Prohibitions and regulations regarding drugs, alcohol, and gambling

An Islāmic perspective

Introduction

The public health approach to addressing alcohol and gambling began in Madinah, Saudi Arabia, 1440 years ago, with Islām establishing a zero-tolerance policy forbidding all intoxicants, including alcohol and gambling. Similarly, responses to excessive drinking emerged in England through the Temperance Society, which opposed alcohol consumption. In the United States, the Eighteenth Amendment to the Constitution in 1918 initiated Prohibition, aiming to halt the trade in alcohol, also known as "The Noble Experiment." The "War on Drugs," particularly notable in the United States, involves government-led efforts to combat illegal drug production, distribution, and consumption through law enforcement measures. Critics argue that this approach has led to high incarceration rates and social inequalities (Fulkerson & Mohammad, 2011). Traditional approaches focusing primarily on legal measures and punitive actions have shown limited success in reducing addiction problems. Addressing addiction requires a more comprehensive strategy involving public health, education, treatment, and addressing underlying social, spiritual, and economic factors contributing to addictive behaviours.

From an Islāmic perspective, the prohibition against intoxicants and gambling is rooted in teachings from the Qur'ân and *hadīth*. Islāmic jurisprudence (the *Shar'iah*), explicitly forbid intoxicants, substances altering one's state of mind, and gambling, deeming them detrimental to spiritual, physical, and mental health. These prohibitions are conveyed through various verses in the Qur'ân revealed over several years. The *hadīth* (sayings of Prophet Muhammad (ﷺ)) emphasising the potential harm they can cause to individuals and society. Scholars often use a holistic approach, considering various Qur'ânic verses and *hadīth*, to derive the principles that guide Islāmic teachings on matters of addiction. The aim of this chapter is to examine the prohibition of intoxicants and gambling from an Islāmic perspective.

DOI: 10.4324/9781032669212-3

Al-khamr

The term *khamr* in the Qur'ān, mentioned six times, equates to liquor in English. Derived from the verb *khamara*, meaning "he covered, hid, or concealed," *khamr* refers to any intoxicating substance that clouds or obscures the intellect. In Islāmic jurisprudence, it encompasses all intoxicants or certain forbidden substances, with its technical definition varying among legal schools. Most jurists, such as those from the Maliki, Shafei's, Hanbali, and *Ahl-i hādīth* schools, interpret it as a general term for any intoxicating beverage made from grapes, dates, or similar substances. However, Hanafi jurists limit the term to grape-based or date-based alcoholic beverages (Campo, 2009), allowing those made with other fruits, grains, or honey. This perspective represents a minority opinion (Ruthven, 1997; Williams, 2020).

It was narrated by 'Umar (may Allāh be pleased with him), "When the prohibition of *khamr* (alcoholic drinks) was revealed, it used to be made from grapes, dates, honey, wheat and barley. *Khamr* is what shields one's mind" (Bulugh al-Maram). The Arabs have different names and attributes of *khamr*. They list about 35 names and the attributes of wine. The Messenger of Allāh (ﷺ) has attributed these names to *khamr* because it symbolises all the following characteristics: *Ummul Khabai'ith*-Fountain (head of evils); *Ummul Fawahish* (The origin of all sorts of atrocities); *Akbarul Kaba'ir* (The most heinous of major sins); *Ra'su Kuli Khatia'* (The head of all errors and lapses); and *Miftahu Kulli Sahrr* (The key to all evils ad mischiefs). The Qur'ān mentions the following types of wine: *Al-khamr, Al-sukr* (Effect of intoxication); and *Al-rahiq* (Clear, pure wine of Paradise).

Qur'ânic perspective on addiction

The earliest Qur'ân verse acknowledges the use of certain fruits, such as dates and grapes, from which people derive both intoxicants and wholesome sustenance. Allāh says in the Qur'ân:

وَمِن ثَمَرَٰتِ ٱلنَّخِيلِ وَٱلْأَعْنَٰبِ تَتَّخِذُونَ مِنْهُ سَكَرًا وَرِزْقًا حَسَنًا ۗ إِنَّ فِى ذَٰلِكَ لَءَايَةٍ لِّقَوْمٍ يَعْقِلُونَ

And from the fruits of palm trees and grapevines, you take intoxicant and good provision. Indeed, in that is a sign for a people who reason.
(An-Nahl 16:67, interpretation of the meaning)

According to the exegesis (*tafsir*) of A'lā al-Mawdūdī, certain fruits, such as dates and grapes, contain both pure and wholesome components as well as substances that can ferment into alcohol when they spoil. The interpretation suggests that individuals have the choice to extract nourishment from these fruits or to indulge in their intoxicating properties, highlighting the presence of both good and evil potentials in certain drinks. Additionally, strong drinks derived from wheat, barley, corn, and honey are also prohibited in Islāmic teachings (Islām Q&A, 2015). Subsequently, a later verse revealed that while alcohol may contain minor benefits, the harm it causes outweighs any potential good. This was the next step in turning people away from consumption of it. Allāh says in the Qur'ân:

وَمِن ثَمَرَٰتِ ٱلنَّخِيلِ وَٱلْأَعْنَٰبِ تَتَّخِذُونَ مِنْهُ سَكَرًا وَرِزْقًا حَسَنًا ۗ إِنَّ فِى ذَٰلِكَ لَءَايَةً لِّقَوْمٍ يَعْقِلُونَ

They ask you about wine and gambling. Say, "In them is great sin and [yet, some](some) benefit for people.

(Al Baqarah 2:219, interpretation of the meaning)

According to the exegesis of Aʿlā al-Mawdūdī, the initial instruction regarding alcoholic drinks and gambling in the Qur'ān involved disapproval rather than an outright prohibition. The Qur'ān acknowledges the potential for some benefit in alcohol but emphasises that its harms, which encompass physical, social, psychological, economic, and spiritual aspects, far outweigh any benefits. Islāmic teachings on intoxicants and gambling are guided by principles aimed at promoting individual and societal well-being while safeguarding individuals from harm. The third mention of alcohol in the Qur'ān appeared as follows:

يَٰٓأَيُّهَا ٱلَّذِينَ ءَامَنُواْ لَا تَقْرَبُواْ ٱلصَّلَوٰةَ وَأَنتُمْ سُكَٰرَىٰ حَتَّىٰ تَعْلَمُواْ مَا تَقُولُونَ

O you who have believe, do not approach prayer when you are intoxicated until you know what you are saying.

(An-Nisā' 4:43, interpretation of the meaning)

This was one of the stages in turning people away from the consumption of alcoholic beverages. Finally, the focus of the rulings was on total abstinence on intoxicants *and* gambling. However, before this last Commandment was given, the Messenger of Allāh (ﷺ)

addressed the people in order to prepare them for its absolute prohibition. He warned and said, "Allāh does not like at all that people should drink wine. Probably absolute prohibition will soon be prescribed: therefore, those who possess wine are advised to sell it."

(Aʿlā al-Mawdūdī)

Finally drinking, gambling, and the like were made absolutely unlawful. Allāh says in the Qur'ân:

يَٰٓأَيُّهَا ٱلَّذِينَ ءَامَنُوٓاْ إِنَّمَا ٱلْخَمْرُ وَٱلْمَيْسِرُ وَٱلْأَنصَابُ وَٱلْأَزْلَٰمُ رِجْسٌ مِّنْ عَمَلِ ٱلشَّيْطَٰنِ فَٱجْتَنِبُوهُ لَعَلَّكُمْ تُفْلِحُونَ

O you who have believed, indeed, intoxicants, gambling, [sacrificing on] stone altars [to other than Allāh], and divining arrows are but defilement from the work of Satan, so avoid it that you may be successful.

(Al-Ma'idah 5: 90, interpretation of the meaning)

إِنَّمَا يُرِيدُ ٱلشَّيْطَـٰنُ أَن يُوقِعَ بَيْنَكُمُ ٱلْعَدَٰوَةَ وَٱلْبَغْضَآءَ فِى ٱلْخَمْرِ وَٱلْمَيْسِرِ وَيَصُدَّكُمْ
عَن ذِكْرِ ٱللَّهِ وَعَنِ ٱلصَّلَوٰةِ ۖ فَهَلْ أَنتُم مُّنتَهُونَ

Satan only wants to cause between you animosity and hatred through intoxicants and gambling and to avert you from the remembrance of Allāh and from prayer. So, will you not desist?

(Al-Mā'idah 5:91, interpretation of the meaning)

A'lā al-Mawdūdī in his *tafsir* (exegesis) posited that in the above verses "Four things have been made absolutely unlawful. They are wine, gambling, ungodly shrines (which are dedicated, to the worship of others than Allāh and in which sacrifices are made and offerings given in the name of others than Allāh) and divining devices." The last verse concludes with a rhetorical question: {Will you not, then, desist?} According to Philips (2008), the grammatical construction used to describe the prohibition of intoxicants in Islāmic texts conveys a strong warning against their consumption. The response of the Prophet's companions highlights the seriousness of the prohibition, emphasising the importance of heeding the warning and taking necessary steps to remove such destructive elements from society. In the Islāmic context, the term "intoxicant" encompasses a range of substances including narcotics, hashish, cannabis, cocaine, morphine, alcohol, and tobacco. Islām unequivocally forbids both intoxicants and gambling, describing them as despicable and hateful acts of Satan. Allāh commands believers to refrain from intoxicants and gambling because they lead to enmity, hostility, and prevent individuals from remembering Allāh.

Hadīth and addiction

The first declaration made by the Prophet (ﷺ) was that not only is *khamr* (wine or alcohol) prohibited but that the definition of *khamr* extends to any substance that intoxicates, in whatever form or under whatever name it may appear. Thus, beer and similar drinks are harām (Shaykh Yusuf Al-Qaradawi, 2001). Ibn 'Umar (may Allāh be pleased with him) narrated that I heard 'Umar while he was on the pulpit of the Prophet (ﷺ) saying,

Now then O people! The revelation about the prohibition of alcoholic drinks was revealed; and alcoholic drinks are extracted from five things: Grapes, dates, honey, wheat, and barley. And the alcoholic drink is that which confuses and stupefies the mind.

(Bukhârî (a))

Prophet Muhammad (ﷺ) stated: "Every intoxicant is *khamr* (wine) and every *khamr* is unlawful" (Ibn Majah (a)). Ibn 'Umar narrated that the Messenger of Allāh (ﷺ) said: "Every intoxicant is *khamr*, and every intoxicant is prohibited" (Muslim). It was narrated that 'Aisha (may Allāh be pleased with her) was asked about drinks and she said: "The Messenger of Allāh (ﷺ) used to forbid all intoxicants" (An-Nasa'i (a)). The Prophet (ﷺ) said, "All drinks that produce intoxication are *harām* (forbidden to drink)" (Bukhârî (b)). It was narrated that Ibn Sirin said: "A man came to Ibn 'Umar and said: "Our families make drinks for us by soaking (fruits) at night, and in the morning we drink them." He said: "I forbid you to drink intoxicants whether in small amounts or large. May Allāh bear witness that I forbid you to drink intoxicants whether in small amounts or large" (An-Nasa'i (b)).

Those Muslims who consume alcohol, no matter what the amount, are breaking the rule and going against the decree set by Allāh. What the individual is doing is unlawful. Abu Hurayrah (may Allāh be pleased with him) narrated that the Prophet (ﷺ) stated:

No one who commits *zina* [adultery and fornication) is a believer at the moment when he is committing *zina*, and no one who drinks wine is a believer at the moment when he is drinking it, and no thief is a believer at the moment when he is stealing, and no killer is a believer at the moment he is killing.

(An-Nasâ'i (c)).

This means that during the time of drinking, he is no longer a believer in the sense of having complete faith. Prophet Muhammad (ﷺ) issued a warning of the punishment in Islām for alcohol drinkers. 'Urwah bin Ruwaim narrated that Ibn Ad-Dailami rode looking for 'Abdullah bin 'Amr bin Al-'As. Ibn Ad-Dailami said:

"I entered upon him and said: 'O 'Abdullah bin 'Amr, did you hear the Messenger of Allāh (ﷺ) say anything concerning *khamr*?' He said: 'Yes, I heard the Messenger of Allāh (ﷺ) say: If a man among my *Ummah* drinks *khamr*, Allāh will not accept his *Salah* [prayer] for forty days" (An-Nasâ'i (d)). What this means is that "he will not be rewarded for them, but he is still obliged to pray; in fact, he is obliged to do all the prayers. If he forsakes prayer during this time, he will be committing one of the worst of major sins, one which some of the scholars said amounts to disbelief, Allāh forbid."

(Islām Q&A, 2002(a))

It was narrated from 'Abdullah bin 'Amr that the Messenger of Allāh (ﷺ) said:

> Whoever drinks wine and gets drunk, his prayer will not be accepted for forty days, and if he dies he will enter Hell, but if he repents, Allāh will accept his repentance. If he drinks wine again and gets drunk, his prayer will not be accepted for forty days, and if he dies he will enter Hell, but if he repents, Allāh will accept his repentance. If he drinks wine again and gets drunk, his prayer will not be accepted for forty days, and if he dies he will enter Hell, but if he repents Allāh will accept his repentance. But if he does it again, then Allāh will most certainly make him drink of the mire of the puss or sweat on the Day of Resurrection.

They said: "O Messenger of Allāh, what is the mire of the pus or sweat? He said: "The drippings of the people of Hell" (Ibn Majah (b)). Prophet Muhammad (ﷺ) also instructed the people to avoid any intoxicating substances whether it intoxicates in a large amount or even when taking in a small amount. "What intoxicates in large amounts, a small amount of it is unlawful" (An-Nasâ'i (e)). For this reason, most observant Muslims avoid alcohol in any form, even small amounts that are sometimes used in cooking.

It is narrated that Ibn 'Umar stated: The Messenger of Allāh (ﷺ) said:

> Wine is cursed from ten angles: The wine itself, the one who squeezes (the grapes etc.), the one for whom it is squeezed, the one who sells it, the one who buys it, the one who carries it, the one to whom it is carried, the one who consumes its price, the one who drinks it and the one who pours it.

(Ibn Majah (c))

It was narrated that Ibn 'Umar (may Allāh be pleased with him) that Prophet Muhammad (ﷺ) stated: "Allāh has cursed wine, its drinker, its server, its seller, its buyer, its presser, the one for whom it is pressed, the one who conveys it, and the one to whom it is conveyed." (Abū Dāwūd). It was narrated from Abu Hurayrah (may Allāh be pleased with him) that the Messenger of Allāh (ﷺ) said: "The one who is addicted to wine is like one who worships idols"(Ibn Majah (d)).

Ibn 'Abbas(may Allāh be pleased with him) reported that the Prophet (ﷺ) said "Whoever dies and has the habit of drinking *khamr*, he will meet Allāh as one who worships idols"(Al-Tabarâni). Ibn 'Umar (may Allāh be pleased with him) reported Allāh's Messenger (ﷺ) as saying: "Every intoxicant is *khamr* and every intoxicant is forbidden. He who drinks wine in this world and dies while he is addicted to it, not having repented, will not be given a drink in the Hereafter" (Muslim (b)). Jabir narrates that a man came from Yemen and asked the Prophet (ﷺ) about a drink that they drank in his homeland that was made of corn and called *Al-mizr* (beer). The Prophet (ﷺ) said to him: "Is it an intoxicant?" He said: "Yes."

It was narrated from Salim bin 'Abdullah that his father said: The Messenger of Allāh (ﷺ) said: "And there are three who will not enter Paradise: The one who disobeys his parents, the drunkard, and the one who reminds people of what he has given them" (An-Nasâ'i (f)). Abu Umâmah (may Allāh be pleased with him) reported that the Messenger of Allāh (ﷺ) said:

> Verily Almighty Allāh sent me as a mercy for all the worlds; and my Almighty and Glorious Lord ordered me to abolish drums, musical instruments, idols, the cross and the affairs of the days of Ignorance. My Almighty and Glorious Lord has sworn, By my honour, no servant among my servants shall drink a mouthful of wine but I will make him drink like it from the scorching water (of hell); and none abstains from it out of fear of me but I will give him drink from the Holy fountain.
>
> (Ahmad (a))

Abu Bakr bin "Abdur-Rahman bin Al-Harith narrated that his father said: who came before you who was a devoted worshipper and used to stay away from people." "And he mentioned something similar. He said: "Avoid *khamr* for, by Allāh, it can never coexist with faith, but soon one of them will expel the other" (An-Nasa'i (h)). The narration emphasises the avoidance of *khamr* (intoxicants, particularly alcoholic beverages) by highlighting that it cannot coexist with faith. This suggests a fundamental incompatibility between engaging in the consumption of intoxicants and maintaining genuine faith. It also highlights the spiritual and moral conflict between indulging in intoxicants and maintaining a strong connection to faith.

From an Islāmic perspective, the underlying principles and prohibitions regarding intoxicants apply to all mind-altering substances, including hashish. Birt (2001) identifies a misconception among certain Muslim users who perceive smoking hashish as less severe than other drugs, often creating an unfounded distinction between hard and soft drugs. The author contends that according to Divine law, all drugs are equally prohibited and fall within the same classification in Islāmic teachings. Islāmic scholars unanimously agree on the prohibition of intoxicating substances, including contemporary drugs. This prohibition is firmly rooted in Islāmic jurisprudence (*Fiqh*), with scholars deriving principles from the Qur'ân and *hādīth* to make judgments on substances unknown at the time of revelation. Philips (2007) asserts that drugs, along with activities like gambling, idolatry, and fortune-telling, are explicitly categorised as prohibited in Islāmic jurisprudence. This alignment stresses the seriousness of the prohibition against intoxicants, including plants with intoxicating properties. The uniform agreement among Islāmic legal schools emphasises that any substance causing intoxication is illegal, extending the prohibition to encompass all intoxicating agents, even those unknown at the time of revelation. This comprehensive stance highlights the Islāmic jurisprudence's firm position against mind-altering substances.

Gambling and games of chance are strongly discouraged and considered a great evil in Islām. Similar to the Qur'ânic verses, the teachings of the Prophet Muhammad (ﷺ) emphasise the prohibition of gambling due to its detrimental effects on individuals and society as a whole. Even the mere consideration of participating in gambling is considered blameworthy in Islām. It has been suggested by the Hanafi scholar Imam Abu Bakr al-Jassas that "There is no difference of opinion between the scholars regarding the prohibition of gambling." (Ahkam al-Qur'ân, 1/329). The Messenger of Allāh (ﷺ) said; "Whoever says to his friend, 'Come, let me gamble with you,' should give something in charity" (Bukhârî (c)).

Muslim users sometimes rationalise tobacco, alcohol, and drug consumption, including *Shisha* smoking, as less serious or even merely disliked (*makrūh*) compared to outright prohibition. This frame of thinking is quite baseless according to Divine law. Muslim scholars are unanimous on the prohibition of contemporary drugs. Sheikh Yusuf Al-Qaradawi (2001), suggested that there is no basis for such differentiation. Islāmic scholars unanimously agree on the prohibition of contemporary drugs, applying principles of Islāmic jurisprudence to derive judgments even on substances unknown during the Qur'anic revelation. Al-Qaradawi emphasises that substances like marijuana, cocaine, and opium fall under the forbidden category of *khamr* due to their ability to distort perception, impair reasoning, and induce escape from reality. This prohibition extends to any recreational drug with similar effects, encompassing cocaine, methamphetamines, heroin, cannabis, and other psychoactive substances. It was narrated from Abu Malik Ash'ari that the Messenger of Allāh (ﷺ)

> People among my nation will drink wine, calling it by another name, and musical instruments will be played for them and singing girls (will sing for them). Allāh will cause the earth to swallow them up and will turn them into monkeys and pigs.
>
> (Ibn Majah (c))

However, there are no prohibitions on using alcohol for scientific, medical, industrial, or automotive use (either as a biofuel, solvent, or a coolant, for instance) (Attar). Abu Bakr bin 'Abdur-Rahman bin Al-Harith narrated that his father said: "I heard 'Uthman say: 'Avoid *khamr* for it is the mother of all evils" (An-Nasâ'i (g)).

Companions of the prophet and scholars' view on addiction

In this section, an overview is provided on the perceptions of the Companions of the Prophet (ﷺ) and classical Muslim scholars on addiction, Ibn Umar (may Allāh be pleased with him) said: I heard Umar (may Allāh be pleased with him) delivering a khutbah [sermon] on the minbar of Madinah and he said: "O people, on the day that the prohibition of *khamr* was revealed, it was made from five things: From grapes, dates, honey, wheat and barley. Khamr is that which overcomes the mind" (An-Nasâ'i (i)). Anas ibn Malik (may Allāh be pleased with him) narrated: I was serving Abu Ubaydah, Abu Talha and Ubay bin Ka'b with a drink prepared from ripe and unripe dates. Then somebody came to them and said, "Alcoholic drinks have been prohibited." (On hearing that) Abu Talha said, "Get up. O Anas and pour (throw) it out! So, I poured (threw) it out. (Bukhârî (d)).

Narrated by Abu Hanifa, Sulayman al-Shaybani reports that Ibn Ziyad (governor of Kufa during the reigns of Mu'awiya I and Yazid I) once told him about an occasion when he was at Ibn Umar's home. The two had been fasting and the time for breaking the fast had come. Ibn Umar offered Ibn Ziyad an alcoholic drink to break his fast with, which his guest duly accepted. Ibn Ziyad became significantly inebriated (*akhadha fihi*). The following morning, having almost not made it back to his home the night before because of the strength of the brew, Ibn Ziyad returned to Ibn Umar to enquire as to the nature of the drink served to him the night before. Ibn Umar explained that he had given his guest no more than dates and raisins (Al-Shaybānī, 2008, pp. 699–700). Ibn Abbas stated "*Khamr* is prohibited for its substance (*bi-ayni-ha*) in small or large quantities in every other beverage" (Al-Ṭaḥāwī, p. 7).

Historical disagreements arose regarding the prohibition of intoxicating drinks in Islāmic jurisprudence. While there was an early consensus against a grape-derived intoxicant, differences persisted on non-grape sources. Various jurists, including Abu Hanifa and others, took differing stances on non-*khamr* intoxicating beverages, leading to a lack of consensus (Sheikh & Islām, 2018). The Maliki School grounded its prohibition arguments in the Qur'ân, while the Shafi'ites focused on Prophetic *hadīths*. Initially, the Hanafi position allowed alcohol consumption beyond *khamr* in moderation, but in the 12th century, they shifted to a more stringent stance, influenced by the reinterpretation of Muhammad al-Shaybānī's views, declaring all intoxicants as prohibited.

Ibn Rushd al-Qurtubi, a Maliki Jurist, stated that

"With respect to *khamr*, [Muslim jurists] are agreed about its prohibition in small or large quantities, I mean, that which is derived from grape juice [...] They agreed that the amount which intoxicates is prohibited. The majority of the jurists of Ḥijāz, as well as the majority of the traditionists, maintained that small and large amounts of intoxicating liquor are prohibited

(Ibn Rushd 2000, p. 571).

According to Sheikh and Islām (2018), "By the expression "Ḥijāzīs", Ibn Rushd refers to the Shāfi'īs, Mālikīs and Hanbalīs; it is worth mentioning that Shiīs and Zaydīs also adopted this position." (p.4)

According to Shaykh al-Islām Ibn Taymiyyah, the prohibition of intoxicants extends beyond substances that cause drunkenness; anything that impairs one's senses is considered haram by the consensus of Muslims (Islām Q&A, 2005). Substances like amphetamine, ecstasy, khat, and heroin, which obstruct the remembrance of Allāh and prayer, are also forbidden. Shaykh Ibn Taymiyyah strongly disapproved of using alcohol for medicinal purposes, emphasising that it is impermissible based on the teachings of the Prophet Muhammad (ﷺ). The Prophet (ﷺ) clarified that alcohol, even for medicinal use, is not a cure but an ailment, and treating diseases with harmful substances is forbidden. Ibn Taymiyyah echoed that

Ibn Masʻood said, "Allāh does not put your cure in that which He has forbidden to you." Ibn Hibbaan (may Allāh have mercy upon him) narrated in his book Sahih Ibn Hibbaan that the Prophet (ﷺ) said, "Allāh does not put the cure for my *Ummah* (community) in that which He has forbidden to them." In addition, it has been narrated that he (ﷺ) was asked about frogs which were used for medicinal purposes. He (ﷺ) forbade killing them and said, "Their croaking is *tasbeeh* (glorification of Allāh)." This is not like consuming dead meat in case of a necessity, for that achieves the purpose of keeping the person alive when he has no alternative; eating it in this case is obligatory, and if a person is forced by necessity to eat dead meat but does not eat it and dies as a result, then he will go to Hellfire. However, in the case of treating disease, the cure is not certain, and this is not the only medicine that one may take; rather, Allāh, The Exalted, may bring about a person's recovery through a variety of means. Moreover, seeking treatment is not obligatory according to the majority of the scholars, so there is no analogy in this case. Allāh knows best.

Ibn al-Qayyim (may Allāh have mercy on him) said:

Treating sickness with unlawful things is abhorrent both from a rational point of view and from an Islāmic point of view. As for the Islāmic point of view, that is seen in the *hadīth* and other texts that we have quoted above. As for reason, that is seen in the fact that Allāh, may He be glorified, only prohibited it because of its evil, for He has not prohibited to this *Ummah* anything good or wholesome as a punishment, as He did in the case of the Children of Israel, as He says [interpretation of the meaning]: For wrongdoing on the part of the Jews, We made unlawful for them [certain] good foods which had been lawful to them [An-Nisa' 4:160]. Rather He prohibited to this *Ummah* what He prohibited because of its evil nature. His prohibition of it is a protection for them, to keep them away from consuming it. So, it is not appropriate to seek healing from sickness and disease by means of it, because even if it could be effective in removing the sickness, that will be followed by sickness that is even worse than it, namely spiritual sickness, because of the strength of its evil nature. Thus, the one who uses it as medicine to remove physical sickness is doing so in a way that causes spiritual sickness. Moreover, the prohibition thereon dictates that one should avoid it and stay away from it by all possible means. Using it as a medicine is making it acceptable to people and making them deal with it, and this is the opposite of what the Lawgiver intended. Moreover, it is a disease, as was stated by the Lawgiver, so it is not permissible to take it as a remedy. Moreover, it will have an impact on man's physical and spiritual being and will cause them to become contaminated with evil because his body will clearly be affected by the evil nature of the remedy. Therefore, if the remedy has evil qualities, it will have an evil impact on his physical being, so how about if the remedy is evil in and of itself? Hence Allāh, may He be glorified, forbade to His slaves all evil foods, drinks and clothing, so that one will not acquire evil qualities under their impact.

(4/141)

The prohibition of alcohol and drugs, according to Philips (2008), involves labelling them as abominations, classifying them with negative activities, attributing a Satanic origin, emphasising avoidance, linking abstinence to success and prosperity, highlighting enmity by sowing discord and hatred, and stressing their role in hindering the remembrance of God and prayer.

Repentance and consequences for addiction

Consuming alcohol or intoxicants is considered *harām* and sin in Islām, and various *hadīths* emphasise that a person engaged in such actions lacks complete faith. It is narrated that Ibn 'Abbas said: "The Messenger of Allāh (ﷺ) said:

No one who commits *zina* [extramarital sexual relations or adultery] is a believer at the moment when he is committing *zina*, and no one who drinks wine is a believer at the moment when he is drinking it, and no thief is a believer at the moment when he is stealing, and no killer is a believer at the moment he is killing.

"(An- Nasâ'i (j))

This means that such a person is not a believer in the sense of having complete faith, rather his faith is greatly lacking because of this evil action. Narrated Ibn `Umar: Allāh 's Messenger (ﷺ) said, "Whoever drinks alcoholic drinks in the world and does not repent (before dying), will be deprived of it in the Hereafter" (Bukhârî (e)).

The punishment for drinking alcohol in this world is flogging, with consensus among scholars. Mu'awiyah narrated that the Messenger of Allāh (ﷺ) said regarding the one who drinks alcohol, "If he drinks (for the first time) flog him, then if he drinks for the second time flog him, then if he drinks for the third time flog him then if he drinks for the fourth time you should kill him" (Ahmad (b). There is a difference in opinion on the number of lashes, with the majority suggesting 80 for a free man and 40 for others. Caliphs Abu Bakr and Umar applied 40 and 80 lashes, respectively, based on consultation with the Prophet's Companions.

The Council of Senior Scholars agrees that the *(hadd)* punishment for drinking wine is 80 lashes **(Islām Q&A**, 2002). Different schools of thought have variations on whether all 80 lashes are punishments or if the second set is a reprimand. According to *Hanafi, Mālikīs and Hanbalīs* lawmen, all of the 80 whips to be hit to the drinker of wine are punishments, whereas the first 40 whips are punishments and the second 40 are reprimand, according to *Shāfi'ī, Zahiri,* and *Zaydi* scholars.

According to scholars such as Ibn Qudamah and Shaykh al-Islam Ibn Taymiyyah, the punishment for drinking alcohol may involve discretion on the part of the Muslim leader. It is suggested that giving more than 40 lashes for the punishment of drinking alcohol is discretionary and lies with the Muslim leader. If the leader deems it necessary, as exemplified during the time of 'Umar, the lashes may be increased to 80. The decision is contingent on the leader's judgement, and Allāh 's knowledge is ultimately supreme (Islām Q&A, 2002). Al-Munajjid (2005) suggested that the punishment for drug consumption aligns with the *(hadd)* punishment for drinking alcohol, as established by Shaykh al-Islam Ibn Taymiyyah, specifically regarding hashish. The reasoning is that drugs, like alcohol, fall under the category of *khamr* and intoxicants, which are explicitly prohibited by Allāh and the Prophet (ﷺ) in Islāmic teachings (Islām Q&A, 2005).

According to Shaykh al-Islam Ibn Taymiyyah, in Islāmic *Shar'iah*, prohibited acts such as drinking wine and engaging in illicit relations incur had punishments. The prescribed punishment for smoking hashish, whether in small or large amounts, is the same as that for drinking wine, which is 80 or 40 lashes. Since hashish is considered a desired substance and renouncing it is challenging for addicts, it is treated similarly to wine, warranting the application of Qur'ânic and *Sunnah* texts related to such prohibited substances. For offenses lacking specified punishments in the Qur'ān or *ḥādīth*, the government may introduce discretionary penalties (*ta'zeer*), such as fines or imprisonment.

References

Abū Dāwūd.) Sunan Abi Dawud 3674. In-book reference: Book 27, Hādīth 6. English translation: Book 26, Hādīth 3666. Sahih (Al-Albani). https://sunnah.com/abudawud:3674

Ahmad. (a). Cited in *The prohibition of intoxicants*. http://Islām.ru/en/content/story/prohibition-intoxicants, (accessed 16 January 2024).

Ahmad. (b). *Bulugh al-Maram*. Book 10, Hadith 41. English translation: Book 10, Hadith 1282. Arabic reference: Book 10, Hadith 1243. https://sunnah.com/bulugh/10/41

Al-Mawdūdī - Sayyid Abul Aᶜlā al-Mawdūdī. *Tafhim al-Qur'an*. http://www.englishtafsir.com/, (accessed 15 January 2024).

Al-Munajjid. (2005). Cited in *Ruling on taking drugs, and do they come under the same heading as khamr (intoxicants)? Fatwa 66227*. https://Islāmqa.info/en/answers/66227/ruling-on-taking-drugs-and-do-they-come-under-the-same-heading-as-khamr-intoxicants, (accessed 16 January 2024).

Al-Shaybānī. (2008). *Kitāb al-āthār*. Kuwait: Dār al-nawādir.

Al-Tabaraani. 12/45; see also Saheeh al-Jaami 6525. Cited in Sheikh Muhammed Salih Al-Munajjid. *Prohibitions that are taken too lightly*. https://Islāmbasics.com/book/prohibitions-that-are-taken-too-lightly/#36,9, accessed 16 January 2024).

Al-Ṭaḥāwī. (2001). *Sharḥ maᶜānī al-āthār*, vol. 4. Beirut: Dar Al-Kotob Al-ilmiyah.

An- Nasâ'i (j). *Sunan an-Nasa'i 4869*. In-book reference: Book 45, Hadith 164. English translation: Vol. 5, Book 45, Hadith 4873. https://sunnah.com/nasai:4869

An-Nasā'i (e). *Sunan an- Nasâ'i 5607*. In-book reference: Book 51, Hādīth 69. English translation: Vol. 6, Book 51, Hādīth 5610. Hasan (Darussalam) https://sunnah.com/nasai:5607. https://sunnah.com/nasai:2562

An-Nasa'i (f). Sunan an-Nasa'i 2562. In-book reference: Book 23, Hādīth 0. English translation: Vol. 3, Book 23, Hādīth 2563. Hasan (Darussalam).

An-Nasa'i (g). *Sunan an-Nasa'i 5667*. In-book reference: Book 51, Hādīth 129. English translation: Vol. 6, Book 51, Hādīth 5670. Sahih (Darussalam). https://sunnah.com/nasai:5667

An-Nasâ'i (a). *Sunan an- Nasâ'i 5682*. In-book reference: Book 51, Hādīth 144. English translation: Vol. 6, Book 51, Hādīth 5685. Sahih (Darussalam). https://sunnah.com/nasai:5682

An-Nasâ'i (b). *Sunan an- Nasâ'i 5581*. In-book reference: Book 51, Hādīth 43. English translation: Vol. 6, Book 51, Hādīth 5584. Sahih (Darussalam). https://sunnah.com/nasai:5581

An-Nasâ'i (c). *Sunan an- Nasâ'i 5682*. In-book reference: Book 51, Hādīth 144. English Translation: Vol. 6, Book 51, Hādīth 5685. Sahih (Darussalam). https://sunnah.com/nasai:5682

An-Nasâ'i (d). *Sunan an- Nasâ'i 5581*. In-book reference: Book 51, Hādīth 43. English translation: Vol. 6, Book 51, Hādīth 5584. Sahih (Darussalam). https://sunnah.com/nasai:5581

An-Nasâ'i (h). *Sunan an-Nasâ'i 5667*. In-book reference: Book 51, Hādīth 129. English translation: Vol. 6, Book 51, Hādīth 5670. Sahih (Darussalam). https://sunnah.com/nasai:5667

An-Nasâ'i (i). *Sunan an-Nasâ'i 5578*. In-book reference: Book 51, Hadith 40. English translation: Vol. 6, Book 51, Hadith 5581. Sahih (Darussalam). https://sunnah.com/nasai:5578

Attar, S. *The alcohol & drug abuse: The American scene and the Islāmic perspective.* https://www.Islāmawareness.net/Alcohol/alcohol_abuse.html, (accessed 16 January 2024).

Birt, Y. (2001). *Being a real man in Islām: Drugs, criminality and the problem of masculinity.* http://masud.co.uk/ISLĀM/misc/drugs.htm, (accessed 16 January 2024).

Bukhârî (a). *Sahih al- Bukhârî* USC-MSA web (English) reference: Vol. 6, Book 60, Hādīth 143. Arabic reference: Book 65, Hādīth 4619.

Bukhârî (b). *Sahih al- Bukhârî 242*. In-book reference: Book 4, Hādīth 109. USC-MSA web (English) reference: Vol. 1, Book 4, Hādīth 243. https://sunnah.com/bukhari:242

Bukhârî (c). Cited in *Fiqh of Gambling.* http://Islāmqa.org/hanafi/daruliftaa/7749, (accessed 16 January 2024).

Bukhârî (d). *Sahih al- Bukhârî 5582*.In-book reference: Book 74, Hadith 8 USC-MSA web (English) reference: Vol. 7, Book 69, Hadith 488. https://sunnah.com/bukhari:5582

Bukhârî (e). *Sahih al- Bukhârî 5575*.In-book reference: Book 74, Hadith 1.USC-MSA web (English) reference: Vol. 7, Book 69, Hadith 481. https://sunnah.com/bukhari:5575

Bulugh al-Maram. Sunnah.com reference: Book 10, Hādīth 46.English translation: Book 10, Hādīth 1286.Arabic reference: Book 10, Hādīth 1247. https://sunnah.com/bulugh/10/46

Campo, J. E. (2009). Dietary rules, in John L. Esposito (Ed.), *The Oxford encyclopaedia of the Islāmic world*. Oxford: Oxford University Press.

Fulkerson, G., & Mohammad, F. (2011). The failure of the war on drugs: A comparative perspective. *Pakistan Journal of Criminology*, 3(2), 55–70.

Ibn Al-Qayyim. *Zaad al-Ma'ad fi Hadiy Khair al-'Ibad*. Cork, Ireland: Sifatu Safwa Corporation.

Ibn Majah (a). *Sunan Ibn Majah 3390*. English reference: Vol. 4, Book 30, Hādīth 3390. Arabic reference: Book 30, Hādīth 3515. Hasan (Darussalam). https://sunnah.com/ibnmajah:3390

Ibn Majah (b). *Sunan Ibn Majah 3377*. In-book reference: Book 30, Hādīth 7. English translation: Vol. 4, Book 30, Hādīth 3377. Sahih (Darussalam). https://sunnah.com/ibnmajah:3377

Ibn Majah (c). *Sunan Ibn Majah 3380*. English reference: Vol. 4, Book 30, Hādīth 3380.Arabic reference: Book 30, Hādīth 3505. Hasan (Darussalam). https://sunnah.com/ibnmajah:3380

Ibn Majah (d). *Sunan Ibn Majah 3375*. English reference: Vol. 4, Book 30, Hādīth 3375. Arabic reference: Book 30, Hādīth 3500. Hasan (Darussalam). https://sunnah.com/ibnmajah:3375

Ibn Majah (e). *Sunan Ibn Majah 4020*. In-book reference: Book 36, Hadith 95. English translation: Vol. 5, Book 36, Hadith 4020. Hasan (Darussalam). https://sunnah.com/ibnmajah:4020

Ibn Rushd. (2000). *The distinguished Jurist's primer Volume 1 Bidāyat al-Mujtahid*, translated by I. A. Khan Nyazee. Reading: Garnet Publishing.

Imam Abu Bakr al-Jassas. Cited in *Fiqh of Gambling*. https://Islāmqa.org/?p=35872, (accessed 16 January 2024).

Islām Q&A. (2002). *What is the punishment for one who drinks alcohol, and are his prayer and fasting valid?* Fatwa 20037. https://Islāmqa.info/en/answers/20037/what-is-the-punishment-for-one-who-drinks-alcohol-and-are-his-prayer-and-fasting-valid, (accessed 16 January 2024).

Islām Q&A. (2005). *Ruling on taking drugs, and do they come under the same heading as khamr (intoxicants)?* Fatwa 66227. https://Islāmqa.info/en/answers/66227/ruling-on-taking-drugs-and-do-they-come-under-the-same-heading-as-khamr-intoxicants, (accessed 16 January 2024).

Muslim (a). *Bulugh al-Maram*. English reference: Book 10, Hādīth 1287. Arabic reference: Book 10, Hādīth 1248. https://sunnah.com/bulugh/10/47

Muslim (b). *Sahih Muslim 2003 a*. In-book reference: Book 36, Hādīth 92. USC-MSA web (English) reference: Book 23, Hādīth 4963. https://sunnah.com/muslim:2003a

Philips, A. A. B. (2007). *The clash of civilizations: An Islāmic view*. Birmingham, UK: Al-Hidaayah Publishing & Distribution.

Philips, A. B. (2008). *War on drugs began 14 centuries ago*. https://ia802203.us.archive.org/15/items/en_War_on_drugs/en_War_on_drugs.pdf, (accessed 15 January 2024).

Ruthven, M. (1997). *Islām: A very short introduction*. Oxford: Oxford University.

Shaykh Ibn Taymiyyah. Cited in Islāmweb.net (2015). *Taking homeopathic medicine that contains alcohol*. Fatwa No: 306379. https://Islāmweb.net/en/fatwa/306379/taking-homeopathic-medicine-that-contains-alcohol, (accessed 16 January 2024).

Shaykh Yusuf Al-Qaradawi. (2001). *The lawful and the prohibited in Islām (Al-Halalwal Haramfil Islām)*. Cairo, Egypt: Al-Falah Foundation for Translation, Publication and Distribution.

Sheikh, M., & Islām, T. (2018). Islām, alcohol, and identity: Towards a critical Muslim studies approach. *ReOrient*, 3(2), 185–211.

Williams, J. A. (2020). *Islām*. Library of Alexandria. E Book.

4 Therapeutic psychosocial and pharmacological interventions

Introduction

The management of addiction requires a holistic approach, considering both physical and psychological aspects of dependence. This includes combining pharmacological detoxification with psychosocial, psycho-educational, and spiritual interventions. Addressing physiological aspects first helps individuals engage better in psychological and spiritual aspects of recovery, enhancing treatment effectiveness and long-term abstinence. Addiction treatment comprises detoxification, maintenance (including substitution or harm-reduction therapies), and abstinence-based therapies. Detoxification focuses on safe substance elimination and withdrawal symptom management, while maintenance therapies aim to minimise harm and reduce relapse risk. Abstinence-based therapies emphasise complete abstinence, using psychological, behavioural, and spiritual interventions. This comprehensive approach tailors strategies to meet the complex needs of addicted individuals seeking treatment. This chapter explores the multifaceted approaches employed to address addictive behaviours, providing an understanding of the intricate interplay between psychological, social, educational, pharmacological strategies, and spirituality.

Overview of pharmacological and behavioural interventions

The initial phase of addiction treatment involves pharmacological detoxification to safely remove addictive substances from the body and manage withdrawal symptoms. Medications like methadone and benzodiazepines may be used for opioid and alcohol addiction, respectively. Following detoxification, psychological interventions address cognitive, emotional, spiritual, and behavioural aspects of addiction. Psychoeducation imparts knowledge about addiction, coping strategies, and stress management. Social interventions rebuild relationships, combat isolation, and foster

DOI: 10.4324/9781032669212-4

healthy connections through support groups and family therapy. Spiritual interventions recognise the role of spirituality, providing individuals with purpose, meaning, and connection, enhancing overall well-being and recovery. Current evidence suggests that pharmaceutical and behavioural treatments can effectively assist clients in reducing alcohol use or achieving abstinence, with addiction treatment demonstrating efficacy in reducing addictive behaviours, improving personal and social functioning, mitigating public health and safety risks, and reducing criminal behaviour (McLellan et al., 1997). Research highlights the significance of medication as a primary approach in treating opioid addiction, often combined with behavioural therapy or counselling, and medications are also effective in addressing alcohol and nicotine addiction. However, for stimulants or cannabis addiction, there are currently no medications available, and treatment relies on behavioural therapies (NIDA, 2023).

Individualised plan in addiction treatment

The management of individuals with addictive behaviours is a multi-faceted task that requires a comprehensive and individualised approach. The complexity of the issues involved often crosses various domains such as medical, psychosocial, social, spiritual, and legal aspects. Thus, intervention strategies must be carefully tailored to address the unique needs of each service user, taking into account the nature and severity of their complex needs. The effectiveness of interventions is closely tied to their appropriateness and the client's readiness to change voluntarily their behaviour and lifestyle. Treatment planning and implementation should be individualised, acknowledging that a one-size-fits-all approach may not be effective. This flexibility allows service providers to adapt interventions based on the unique circumstances and progress of each client.

Developing an individualised plan in addiction treatment is essential for addressing the unique needs of each person. Key components include a comprehensive assessment, client-centred goals, tailored treatment modalities, consideration of medical and psychosocial factors, relapse prevention strategies, a holistic approach, and addressing legal and vocational aspects. Addressing underlying issues such as mental health conditions or dual diagnosis (Rassool, 2001) and trauma is essential for long-term success. Ongoing assessment, clear communication, and flexibility to adjust the plan as needed are crucial for enhancing the effectiveness of addiction treatment and promoting successful recovery. This client- centred and flexible approach ensures that the intervention strategies align with the specific needs and readiness of the individual, promoting a more responsive and tailor-made treatment strategy and the therapeutic journey.

Detoxification and management of withdrawal

Detoxification, or detox, is the initial phase in treating substance use disorders, involving the safe management of withdrawal symptoms when an individual stops using alcohol or drugs. Key principles include medical supervision, thorough assessment, individualised plans, pharmacotherapy to alleviate withdrawal symptoms, continuous monitoring, emotional support, nutritional care, and education about the detoxification process.

The role of detoxification acts as a preliminary step before implementing social and psychological interventions. It is aimed at influencing and motivating the service users to change their behaviours (Gafoor & Rassool, 1998). Medically assisted detoxification can be delivered both in the community and in hospital settings. Community or home detoxification is based on the principle that the service users remain in their own natural environment, and this approach is rooted in social learning theory (Gafoor & Rassool, 1998; Davis, 2018). This is based on the premise that drinking is a learned behaviour in response to environmental and social cues. Additionally, it notes that individuals with a history of severe alcohol withdrawal symptoms like fits or delirium tremens may necessitate hospital detoxification, highlighting the importance of considering the severity of withdrawal symptoms in determining the appropriate care setting. Alcohol, opiates, and hypno-sedatives can lead to significant physical withdrawal symptoms, requiring pharmacological treatments to alleviate withdrawal effects. The alcohol withdrawal syndrome typically spans about 5 days, with the highest risk of severe withdrawal occurring in the initial 24 to 48 hours. While opiate withdrawal is usually not life-threatening, withdrawal from alcohol and hypno-sedatives poses notable risks, including a significant mortality and morbidity rate, without appropriate pharmacological interventions. A comprehensive account of the withdrawal signs and symptoms of psychoactive substances is found in Rassool (2025).

Pharmacological interventions

Effective pharmacological treatment in addiction involves tailored medications to address specific consequences of substance or behavioural addiction. However, pharmacological interventions are not standalone and are recommended alongside psychosocial therapies (O'Brien & McKay, 2007; Raistrick et al., 2003; Woody, 2003). The goal is harm reduction, using medications like methadone for opiate users, managing withdrawal symptoms, maintaining abstinence, preventing relapse, and addressing co-existing substance misuse and psychiatric disorders (dual diagnosis). Pharmacological interventions aim to enhance overall well-being and support recovery from addictive behaviours. The primary goals of pharmacological interventions in alcohol withdrawal are outlined as follows: to alleviate subjective withdrawal symptoms, prevent and manage more severe complications, and prepare individuals for subsequent structured psychosocial and educational interventions (Rassool, 2018, 2025).

Alcohol addiction: Pharmacological interventions

Pharmacological interventions play a significant role in the treatment of alcohol addiction. In alcohol use disorder (AUD) treatment, three medications provide diverse strategies: disulfiram ensures compliance; naltrexone reduces alcohol reward and craving; acamprosate lessens post-alcohol excitability. The American Psychiatric Association (APA, 2018) recommends naltrexone or acamprosate for individuals with moderate to severe AUD aiming to reduce alcohol consumption or achieve abstinence. Disulfiram is suggested for those pursuing abstinence, while topiramate or gabapentin are options for reducing alcohol consumption. In the United Kingdom, the National Institute for Health and Care Excellence (NICE) (2011) advocates a stepped approach to treating AUD, starting with motivational interviewing (MI) and psychological interventions like cognitive-behavioural therapy. For non-responsive cases, acamprosate or oral naltrexone may be integrated. This treatment extends to comorbid psychosis and substance use disorder (dual diagnosis), with antipsychotic medications added when necessary. No specific drug is approved for dual diagnosis populations, but medications are generally considered viable, except for disulfiram (Pharmaceutical Press, 2013). To expedite the detoxification process, minor tranquillisers such as chlordiazepoxide or diazepam are commonly employed. Diazepam, in particular, is noted for its anti-convulsant effects, providing a safeguard against seizures during the withdrawal period. It is important to note that pharmacological interventions in AUD may vary based on individual needs, medical history, and potential interactions with other medications.

Acamprosate

Acamprosate is a medication used to support individuals in maintaining abstinence from alcohol. It influences neurotransmitters in the brain. Side effects may include diarrhoea, nausea, and insomnia. Administered orally for several months, it forms part of a comprehensive treatment plan with psychosocial interventions (APA, 2018). Typically administered orally, acamprosate is prescribed for several months as part of a comprehensive treatment plan that includes psychosocial interventions.

Naltrexone

Naltrexone is used to treat alcohol and opioid dependence. It functions as an opioid receptor antagonist (substance that opposes or blocks the action of another substance in the body), blocking the effects of opioids in the brain. This helps reduce cravings and the rewarding effects of alcohol and opioids. Naltrexone is used in both oral and injectable forms, providing a monthly dose. Common side effects include nausea, headache, dizziness, and fatigue. Adherence to the prescribed treatment plan is crucial for effectiveness.

Disulfiram

Disulfiram is used for the treatment of AUD by creating an aversion to alcohol consumption. It inhibits the enzyme acetaldehyde dehydrogenase, leading to the accumulation of toxic acetaldehyde when alcohol is consumed. This results in unpleasant symptoms, such as flushing and nausea, aiming to deter individuals from drinking. Common side effects include drowsiness and a metallic taste. Supervised administration may be considered to ensure compliance and monitor for adverse reactions.

Thiamine deficiency

Wernicke–Korsakoff syndrome is a neurological disorder resulting from thiamine (vitamin B1) deficiency, often associated with AUD. It comprises Wernicke's encephalopathy, an acute condition with confusion and eye movement abnormalities, and Korsakoff syndrome, a chronic state marked by severe memory impairment. Thiamine supplementation, especially through parenteral administration in severe cases, is crucial for treatment and prevention (NICE, 2010). In individuals undergoing planned and assisted alcohol withdrawal, prophylactic thiamine is recommended, emphasising the importance of nutritional support and early intervention to prevent irreversible neurological consequences of alcohol addiction.

Opiate and opioids addiction: Pharmacological interventions

Detoxification for opiate users involves the process of safely removing opiates from the body while managing withdrawal symptoms. Opiate detoxification can occur in various settings, including outpatient clinics, rehabilitation centres, or hospitals, depending on the severity of addiction and individual needs. Medications may be prescribed to alleviate withdrawal symptoms and reduce cravings. Common medications used for opiate detoxification include methadone, buprenorphine (Suboxone), and naltrexone. The duration of opiate detoxification can vary depending on several factors, including the individual's level of opiate dependence, the specific opiates used, the method of detoxification, and the presence of any co-occurring medical or mental health conditions. In general, opiate detoxification can last anywhere from a few days to a couple of weeks. Opiate detoxification duration varies depending on the individual, typically lasting up to 28 days as an inpatient or up to 12 weeks as an outpatient. Users ready to discontinue maintenance opioid substitution therapy (OST) can opt for detoxification. Some may choose detoxification upon starting treatment (Public Health England, 2021).

Methadone opiate addiction

Methadone treatment is a primary approach for managing opiate addiction globally (Kreek & Vocci, 2002). It offers controlled symptom relief over an extended period when taken orally once a day, suppressing withdrawal for 24–36 hours. Methadone is effective for opiate use disorder but not suitable for other substances. It is recommended for individuals with a history of relapse and treatment drop-out. Methadone maintenance treatment provides individualised healthcare and prescribed methadone to alleviate withdrawal, reduce cravings, and establish biochemical balance. By blocking heroin's euphoric effects, methadone diminishes cravings and aids detoxification. Extended therapy may be necessary without adverse effects, implying physical dependence but returning positive outcomes. Methadone maintenance offers stability and relief from challenges associated with opiate addiction, facilitating functional lives.

Methadone treatment begins with a baseline dose to alleviate withdrawal symptoms and minimise overdose risk, with individualised dose reductions based on assessments and treatment plans. Reductions can occur rapidly (7–21 days) or slowly over several months, with higher initial doses allowing for greater reduction. The process should be gradual, Subatnce Abusewconsidering factors like anxiety and the individual's sense of control, with varied reduction intervals and psychological support as needed. Regular monitoring and multidisciplinary team discussions are crucial. Methadone maintenance treatment has shown positive outcomes, including reduced illicit drug consumption and criminal behaviour, and lower HIV risk behaviours and seroconversion rates (Sorensen & Copeland, 2000; Gossop et al., 2002; Teoh Bing Fei et al., 2016). However, it may not effectively reduce sex-related HIV risk-taking behaviour (Teoh Bing Fei et al., 2016).

Naltrexone

Naltrexone, a long-acting opioid antagonist, is primarily used to manage opiate addiction, distinct from naloxone used in emergency overdose cases. It prevents relapse by blocking euphoric effects of opiates, hindering a return to physical dependence. It can be administered orally or as an implant with minimal adverse effects. Naltrexone is ideal for individuals in early addiction stages and highly motivated for treatment. While its use in relapse prevention shows minor positive effects, it provides almost ideal treatment for opiate addiction, potentially alleviating discomfort during withdrawal and preventing relapse (Sing & Saadabadi, 2023). Naltrexone, administered orally or as an implant, minimises adverse effects and blocks the euphoric effects of opiates like heroin, preventing a return to physical dependence. It is suitable for individuals in early addiction stages and highly motivated for treatment. However, its clinical management of heroin addiction has limitations due to its limited impact, costliness, and client resistance (NTA, 2006). Naltrexone can cause serious side effects, including risk of opioid overdose, severe reactions at the site of the naltrexone injection (injection site reactions), sudden opioid withdrawal, and liver damage or hepatitis (Thornton, 2023). There is a need for caution when naltrexone is used in the treatment of addiction, since many addicts have liver disease associated with viral hepatitis infections (NTA, 2006).

Buprenorphine

Buprenorphine, a partial opiate agonist, provides an alternative to methadone in reducing cravings and withdrawal symptoms while having a lower risk of abuse and overdose compared to full agonists. Buprenorphine is a medication used in the treatment of opioid dependence, functioning as a partial opioid agonist. It binds to opioid receptors, reducing withdrawal symptoms and cravings without causing intense euphoria. Administered daily as a sublingual tablet, buprenorphine binds to opioid receptors, lessening withdrawal symptoms and cravings without intense euphoria. Compared to methadone, it produces lower euphoric effects, resulting in less euphoria, physical dependence, and misuse potential. Buprenorphine also causes milder withdrawal symptoms and is safer in overdose due to limited respiratory depression effects. It is viewed as an alternative to methadone maintenance with an effective duration of at least 24 hour and is effective in managing opioid withdrawal. However, this medication for detoxification can worsen withdrawal symptoms if used in combination with methadone or other opioids.

Non-opiate treatments

Non-opiate treatments, such as lofexidine, are now available for opiate withdrawal, offering effectiveness in symptom alleviation without the risk of client misuse Lofexidine, a fully licensed drug in the United Kingdom for managing opiate withdrawal symptoms, can be supervised in various settings, including inpatient, residential, and community settings

(Department of Health, 1999). The US Food and Drug Administration has approved the use of lofexidine for alleviating withdrawal symptoms to facilitate the abrupt cessation of opioids in adults. Lofexidine has been shown to be effective in reducing withdrawal symptoms and renewed cravings (Urits et al., 2020). Clonidine is not licensed for the treatment of opiate withdrawal symptoms but is useful as a non-opiate treatment for opiate withdrawal. It can provide relief to many of the physical symptoms of opioid withdrawal including sweating, diarrhoea, vomiting, abdominal cramps, chills, anxiety, insomnia, and tremor (WHO, 2009).

Pharmacological interventions for other addictions

For nicotine addiction nicotine replacement therapy significantly increases smoking cessation rates. Bupropion, an antidepressant, also enhances smoking abstinence rates.

High-certainty evidence suggests that bupropion can aid long-term smoking cessation. However, bupropion also increases the occurrence of adverse events, including psychiatric adverse events (Howes et al., 2020). Additionally, there is high-certainty evidence indicating that individuals taking bupropion are more likely to discontinue treatment compared to those taking a placebo. Novel agents like rimonabant and varenicline show promising results. Rimonabant acts by blocking cannabinoid receptors in the brain, reducing the rewarding effects of nicotine, while varenicline targets nicotine receptors, reducing nicotine cravings and withdrawal symptoms, thus aiding in quitting smoking. These medications offer additional options for individuals seeking to quit smoking. For gambling disorder, there is available evidence, of low-quality, that suggests that opioid antagonists and antipsychotics, but not antidepressants, may be effective in reducing the severity of gambling symptoms (Dowling et al., 2022). The authors suggested that there is insufficient information to determine their impact on other gambling and psychological symptoms, and the effectiveness of mood stabilisers remains uncertain.

Psychosocial interventions

Psychosocial interventions aim to enhance the psychosocial well-being of individuals struggling with addiction. These encompass various approaches including brief interventions, psychotherapy, counselling, MI, motivational enhancement therapy, solution-focused therapy, community reinforcement approach, social behaviour and network therapy, coping and social skills training, marital therapy, relapse prevention, and complementary therapies. Guidelines issued by NICE (2007a, 2007b) provide comprehensive recommendations on psychosocial interventions for adults and young people misusing opioids, cannabis, or stimulants. A fundamental principle of good practice in psychological interventions involves assessing the health and social care needs of individuals to guide appropriate intervention types. Key working, involving regular contact between service providers and clients, is crucial, serving as a basic delivery mechanism for various psychosocial components. Interventions include regular reviews of care plans and treatment goals, offering advice and information on alcohol and drug misuse, harm reduction strategies, motivational enhancements, relapse prevention, and addressing social problems like family issues, housing, and employment. The effectiveness of the therapeutic alliance is paramount for successful treatment delivery and positive client outcomes. Treatment goals should be mutually agreed upon between the key worker and the client, ensuring a client-directed approach.

Brief interventions

Brief interventions aim to motivate individuals at risk of alcohol and substance use disorder to change their behaviour. The goal is to help clients recognise the risks associated with alcohol or drug use and encourage them to reduce or cease substance use. According to the World Health Organization, brief interventions are strategies to identify existing or potential issues related to substance use, with the primary objective of motivating individuals to modify their substance use behaviour (Henry-Edwards et al., 2003). These interventions operate on the harm reduction principle, aiming to help individuals understand the problems associated with their substance abuse patterns and initiate behaviour modification to reduce harms caused by substance use (Sarkar et al., 2020). Brief interventions can be a single brief advice session or several short counselling sessions lasting 15–30 minutes. They are not meant for individuals with alcohol or substance use disorder but are aimed at those engaging in problematic or risky substance use. Brief interventions may motivate individuals with more serious dependence to consider more intensive treatment within primary care or seek specialised alcohol and drug services. Screening tools facilitate the identification of intervention targets, highlighting individuals consuming substances at hazardous levels (Heather & Kaner, 2001).

The acronym "FRAMES" condenses the key elements of effective brief interventions, as outlined by Bien et al. (1993). These elements are **F**eedback, **R**esponsibility, **A**dvice, **M**enu, **E**mpathy, and **S**elf-efficacy. Brief interventions, characterised by their positive and supportive approach, can be effectively delivered by health or social services workers in a non-judgmental manner. Table 4.1 depicts the elements of brief interventions.

Table 4.1 Elements of effective brief interventions

	Acronym	Elements	Therapeutic responses
F	Feedback	Feedback of personal risk or impairment	Your punctuality issues at work might be linked to your alcohol or drug usage.Sharing of results of assessments such as cognitive testing and liver function tests to provide insights into potential connections between substance use and workplace challenges.
R	Responsibility	Emphasis on personal responsibility for change	The responsibility for deciding to quit substance misuse for the next two weeks lies with you.
A	Advice	A clear advice to change	A recommendation is made for you to refrain from drinking or drug use for the next two weeks to assess if this change has a positive impact.
M	Menu	Menu of alternative change options	If you find it challenging to reduce or stop your substance misuse, alternative options, such as alcoholics anonymous (AA) or narcotics anonymous (NA), or referral to a specialist service, are suggested.
E	Empathy	Therapeutic empathy as a counselling style	Acknowledging that abstaining from alcohol might be challenging for you, especially considering its role in helping you to relax after a stressful working day.
S	Self-Efficacy	Enhancement of patient self-efficacy or optimism	Recognising the challenges you face; I am confident in your abilities and strengths to contemplate changing your behaviour.

Source: Adapted from Rassool (2018).

The NICE (2007b) guideline on psychosocial interventions recommends offering opportunistic brief interventions, focused on motivation, to individuals with limited contact with drug services, such as those attending needle and syringe exchanges or primary care settings, especially when concerns about substance use disorder are identified. These brief interventions typically involve two sessions, each lasting 10–45 minutes, aimed at exploring ambivalence about substance use, increasing motivation for behavioural change, and providing non-judgmental feedback. Additionally, NICE (2007b) suggests that service providers routinely offer information about self-help groups based on 12-step principles, including well-known groups like alcoholics anonymous (AA), narcotics anonymous (NA), and cocaine anonymous (CA), to individuals who misuse drugs. This comprehensive approach to addressing addiction utilises motivational interventions and encourages additional support through participation in self-help groups. The alcohol, smoking and substance involvement screening test (ASSIST), developed by the World Health Organization (WHO, 2002), identifies psychoactive substance use and related problems in primary care clients. ASSIST is a valid screening test for identifying substance use in individuals who use multiple substances and have varying degrees of use (Humeniuk et al., 2008). A manual has been developed for primary care use (Humeniuk et al., 2012).

The use of a self-help manual has been identified as more effective than minimal advice alone. Research studies highlight that any form of brief intervention, even if relatively minimal, is preferable to providing no therapeutic intervention at all (Heather et al., 1986; Heather, 1998). A recent Cochrane review by Kaner et al. (2018), encompassing 69 studies and over 33,000 participants, found that brief interventions led to reduced alcohol consumption compared to minimal or no intervention participants after one year. This effect was observed for both men and women. However, the review found that brief interventions had a statistically significant but minimal impact on the frequency of binge drinking and drinking days per week.

Psychotherapy, counselling, and motivational interviewing

Psychotherapy and counselling play a vital role in addiction treatment, addressing the psychological aspects of addiction. Various approaches are employed, including cognitive-behavioural therapy (CBT) for changing thought patterns, MI to enhance motivation, mindfulness-based approaches for self-awareness, psychodynamic therapy to explore root causes, dialectical behaviour therapy (DBT) for emotion management, 12-step facilitation therapy for community engagement, family therapy for interpersonal dynamics, and trauma-informed therapy for addressing past trauma.

The therapeutic process begins with a comprehensive assessment of the substance user's needs, emphasising the maintenance of rapport through qualities like empathy, genuineness, and a non-judgemental approach. Recognising and highlighting positive aspects related to addiction can enhance an individual's self-efficacy and self-esteem, reducing resistance to engaging with services and fostering effective coping strategies and treatment outcomes. Acknowledging strengths involves identifying successful past strategies and drug-free coping mechanisms, contributing to an empowering therapeutic process (Rassool, 2006, 2025). Velleman (2011) proposes a six-stage counselling approach for individuals with substance use disorder, emphasising trust development, problem exploration, goal setting, empowerment for action, support in maintaining changes, and mutual agreement on the conclusion of the therapeutic relationship. The effectiveness of therapy is closely tied to the alignment of therapeutic techniques with a client's goals. No single approach is universally suitable, emphasising the importance of tailoring methods to individual needs.

MI is employed when clients exhibit little or no commitment to change. Defined by Rollnick and Miller (1995), MI is a directive yet client-centred therapy aiming to induce behavioural change by enabling clients to explore and resolve ambivalence. This approach involves actively guiding clients to examine motivations and uncertainties to facilitate positive behaviour changes. MI operates under the assumption that deficient motivation is the primary barrier to altering addictive behaviours and related patterns, with enhancing motivation becoming crucial for increasing the likelihood of behavioural change (Baker & Reicher, 1998). MI has been widely and effectively utilised in individuals dealing with addiction issues, aiming to enhance engagement and reduce substance use (Miller & Rollnick, 2013). This technique is accessible without requiring extensive psychotherapy or counselling knowledge and involves a non-judgemental approach, open-ended questioning, and reflective listening. Its purpose is to elevate the client's self-esteem, self-efficacy, and awareness of their problems. MI elicits self-motivational statements from the client, emphasising their motivated behaviour while highlighting that the responsibility for change lies with the client. The four key principles of MI include expressing empathy, developing discrepancy, rolling with resistance, and supporting self-efficacy.

Various tools and strategies, including pencil and paper exercises, structured questions, and focused reflections, have been developed to implement the principles of MI. The findings of a Cochrane review (Schwenker et al., 2023) indicate that MI may have limited impact on substance use disorder when compared to standard treatment or another active intervention. In the short term, it appears to be more effective in reducing substance use when compared to no treatment. However, at medium- and long-term follow-up, MI likely leads to a slight reduction in substance use compared with assessment and feedback. The impact of MI on willingness to change and treatment retention remains unclear.

Contingency management

Contingency management (CM), rooted in operant conditioning principles, offers incentives like vouchers or prize draws to individuals in addiction treatment for achieving positive outcomes, such as clean drug tests or maintaining sobriety, while withholding incentives if goals are not met

(NIDA, 2020). NICE recommends incorporating CM programmes in drug services to reduce illicit drug use and improve engagement, especially for those in methadone maintenance treatment (NICE, 2007b). Research indicates that CM effectively increases treatment retention, medication compliance, and promotes abstinence from drugs and alcohol (SAMHSA, 2020). Strong evidence supports CM's use in reducing stimulant use like methamphetamine or cocaine (SAMHSA, 2021), with benefits extending to individuals addicted to opioids, alcohol, marijuana, and benzodiaze-pines, as reported in various studies showing positive outcomes (SAMHSA, 2020, 2021).

Cue exposure therapy

Cue exposure therapy (CET) is a behavioural therapy technique used in addiction treatment to reduce the impact of triggers or cues that can induce cravings and lead to relapse. Childres et al. (1988) identified that repetitive associations between substance use and specific cues, such as settings, indi-viduals, emotional states, and paraphernalia, could result in significant conditioned craving. They demonstrated "cue reactivity," indicating both physiological responses (changes in skin temperature) and subjective responses (withdrawal-like symptoms, craving) in individuals with opiate and cocaine dependencies when exposed to drug-related stimuli, such as handling drug paraphernalia. CET involves exposing individuals with drug or alcohol use issues to cues associated with addiction, aiming to diminish the desire to use substances. It has the potential to reduce cravings trig-gered by specific cues, allows practising coping responses, and enhances self-efficacy. CET shows promise as an alcohol treatment method with ben-efits comparable to other effective psychosocial treatments (Byrne et al., 2019). However, findings from a randomised controlled trial by Marissen et al. (2007) suggest that CET, compared to non-specific psychotherapy, may lead to higher dropout and relapse rates among abstinent heroin-dependent individuals in a drug-free setting. This indicates caution should be exer-cised when considering the application of CET in this specific context.

Relapse prevention

Relapse prevention is a cognitive-behavioural technique focused on teach-ing coping skills to individuals grappling with addiction. It involves iden-tifying situations where coping inadequacies occur and utilising methods such as instruction, modelling, role-plays, and behavioural rehearsal. Gradual exposure to stressful situations is implemented as adaptive mas-tery occurs. A relapse prevention plan, based on identified risk factors, includes elements like assertiveness work and social inclusion. Training in relapse prevention skills covers reducing substance exposure, evaluating the pros and cons of continued use, self-monitoring for high-risk situations, developing strategies for coping with cravings, identifying risky thought processes, preparing for emergencies, and completing homework assignments. Relapse prevention shows promise in reducing relapse severity, extending treatment effects' durability, and proving beneficial for clients with dependence severity (Carroll, 1996). There is substantial evidence supporting the effectiveness of specific relapse prevention in dealing with high-risk situations for alcohol use (Sharma et al., 2022).

Marital and family therapies

Marital and family therapies (MFT) in addiction treatment focus on understanding and addressing family dynamics. These therapies explore the role of significant others in the addictive process, identify sources of stress related to addiction, and help families develop more effective coping behaviours. Issues within marital relationships, such as poor communication and problem-solving skills, can precede harmful substance use and contribute to relapse. The National Institute of Clinical Excellence Guidelines (NICE, 2011) recommends behavioural couples therapy specifically for individuals dealing with harmful drinking and alcohol dependence. MFT, including behavioural couples therapy (BCT), has shown effectiveness in alcohol treatment and reducing dropout and relapse rates (Fals-Stewart & Birchler, 2001; Moyers & Hester, 1999; NICE, 2007b, 2011).

Traditional, Minnesota model, 12-step-oriented model

Rooted in the perspective of addiction as both a spiritual and medical disease, approaches like AA offer mutual support for individuals striving to maintain sobriety. AA, established in the United States in 1933, has expanded globally, spawning groups like NA for drug users, and Al-Anon and families anonymous (FA) for affected families. AA groups provide regular meetings in various settings, fostering group identity, open confession, and confidential sharing among members. AA is explicitly spiritual, not religious, welcoming individuals with diverse beliefs. For those without comorbid conditions, 12-step programmes show high effectiveness in long-term abstinence, with recent evidence supporting their efficacy (Laudet et al., 2004; Greene, 2021). However, dropout rates from 12-step programs remain a concern (Lilienfeld & Arkowitz, 2011).

Social interventions

The social model emphasises the interplay between an individual's internal experiences and their external social environments, networks, and communities. Recognising the significant role families can play in substance use disorder treatment, interventions based on this model empower and support individuals and their family social networks in developing coping strategies for social problems. Family involvement can impact the prevention and course of substance misuse issues, improve outcomes for the user, and mitigate negative effects on other family members (Copello et al., 2006). Addressing issues like housing and childcare through advocacy can directly influence an individual's ability to address substance misuse. Robust evidence supports the effectiveness of family-focused and social network-focused interventions, often returning outcomes equal to or better than individual interventions. This approach underscores the importance of considering the broader social context in addiction treatment.

Complementary therapies

Complementary therapies in addiction treatment encompass non-traditional or alternative approaches used alongside conventional methods to enhance overall recovery. Auricular acupuncture, pioneered by Dr. Wen in 1972, has shown promise in relieving opioid withdrawal symptoms (Cui et al., 2008). This therapy has been applied to various substance use disorder and addictive behaviours, including AUD, methadone detoxification, opiate detoxification, cocaine, crack cocaine, and tobacco addiction, as well as preventing relapse. The limited adoption of acupuncture detoxification therapy is attributed not only to a lack of understanding of its physiological mechanisms but also to the scarcity of controlled clinical studies and a failure to describe acupuncture in quantitative Western terms (Katims et al., 1992). The efficacy of acupuncture in detoxification treatment remains largely anecdotal, and despite its utilisation in certain clinics and drug court programmes, acupuncture is still considered an alternative medicine (Spray & Jones, 1995). Evaluations of the NADA protocol in addiction treatment have shown mixed results, ranging from promising early randomised controlled trials to a combination of positive and negative studies (Stuyt & Voyles, 2016). While National Acupuncture Detoxification Association (NADA) is not a standalone procedure but a psychosocial intervention impacting the whole person, it has the potential to be a complementary tool in the detoxification process. However, a randomised controlled trial by Ahlberg et al. (2016) investigating the effects of auricular acupuncture on anxiety, sleep, drug use, and utilisation of addiction treatment services found no evidence supporting the superiority of acupuncture over relaxation. The study revealed no significant effectiveness of acupuncture in addressing issues related to anxiety, sleep problems, substance use, or reducing the necessity for additional addiction treatment in individuals with coexisting psychiatric disorders.

Aromatherapy utilises natural essences from aromatic plants to facilitate healing for the body, mind, and spirit, with essential oils possessing unique properties obtained through distillation and extraction. Administered by qualified practitioners due to contraindications, aromatherapy, particularly when combined with massage, can offer stress relief and relaxation in addiction treatment (McDonald & Rassool, 1997). While generally welcomed by clients, there is limited literature on its use in addiction treatment. Advocates like Miller and Walker (1997) suggest that therapeutic interventions should be available until proven ineffective or harmful. Reflexology, a complementary treatment for addiction, involves practitioners working on the feet or hands to identify imbalances and energy blockages, applying compression massage techniques to specific areas. Beyond physical benefits, clients often experience relaxation in a secure environment, contributing to healing on physical, psychological, and emotional levels. However, evidence supporting reflexology's efficacy in various conditions remains limited, except for potential relief of urinary symptoms in multiple sclerosis (Wang et al., 2008).

Complementary therapies provide valuable options in addiction services due to their cost-effectiveness and generally low therapeutic risks. However, further research is necessary to evaluate their safety and effectiveness fully. Establishing appropriate professional and legal regulations is crucial to ensure their proper use. Additionally, some complementary therapies may not be suitable for specific communities due to conflicting belief systems.

References

Ahlberg, R., Skårberg, K., Brus, O., & Kjellin, L. (2016). Auricular acupuncture for substance use: A randomized controlled trial of effects on anxiety, sleep, drug use and use of addiction treatment services. *Substance Abuse Treatment, Prevention, and Policy*, 11(1), 24. https://doi.org/10.1186/s13011-016-0068-z

American Psychiatric Association. (2018). *The American Psychiatric Association practice guideline for the pharmacological treatment of clients with alcohol use disorder*. Washington, D.C: American Psychiatric Association Publishing. https://doi.org/10.1176/appi.books.9781615371969

Baker, A., & Reicher, R. (1998). Motivational interviewing. *Clinical skills series. Effective approaches to alcohol and other drug problems*. Suffolk: Visual Education.

Bien, T.H., Miller, W.R., & Tonigan, J.S. (1993) Brief interventions for alcohol problems: A review. *Addiction*, 88, 315–336.

Byrne, S. P., Haber, P., Baillie, A., Giannopolous, V., & Morley, K. (2019). Cue exposure therapy for alcohol use disorders: What can be learned from exposure therapy for anxiety disorders? *Substance Use & Misuse*, 54(12), 2053–2063. https://doi.org/10.1080/10826084.2019.1618328

Carroll, K. M. (1996). Relapse prevention as a psychosocial treatment: A review of controlled clinical trials. *Experimental and Clinical Psychopharmacology*, 4(1), 46–54.

Childres, A. R., McLellan, A. T., Ehrman, R., & O'Brien, C. P. (1988). Classically conditioned responses in opioid and cocaine dependence: A role in relapse?, in B. A. Ray (Ed.), *Learning factors in substance abuse* (DHHS Publication No. 88-1576). Washington, DC: U.S. Government Printing Office, pp. 25–43.

Copello, A. G., Templeton, L., & Velleman, R. (2006). Family interventions for drug and alcohol misuse: Is there a best practice? *Current Opinion in Psychiatry*, 19(3), 271–276.

Cui, C. L., Wu, L. Z., & Luo, F. (2008). Acupuncture for the treatment of drug addiction. *Neurochemical Research*, 33(10), 2013–2022. https://doi.org/10.1007/s11064-008-9784-8

Davis, C. (2018). Home detox – supporting clients to overcome alcohol addiction. *Australian Prescriber*, 41(6), 180–182. https://doi.org/10.18773/austprescr.2018.059

Department of Health. (1999). *Drug misuse and dependence – Guidelines on clinical management*. London: The Stationery Office.

Dowling, N., Merkouris, S., Lubman, D., Thomas, S., Bowden-Jones, H., & Cowlishaw, S. (2022). Pharmacological interventions for the treatment of disordered and problem gambling. *Cochrane Database of Systematic Reviews*, 2022(9), Art. No. CD008936. https://doi.org/10.1002/14651858.CD008936.pub2

Fals-Stewart, W., & Birchler, G. R. (2001). A national survey of the use of couples therapy in substance abuse treatment. *Journal of Substance Abuse Treatment*, 20(4), 277–286. https://doi.org/10.1016/s0740-5472(01)00165-9

Gafoor, M., & Rassool, G. Hussein. (1998). Alcohol: Community detoxification and clinical care, in G. Hussein Rassool (Ed.), *Substance use and misuse: Nature, context and clinical interventions*. Oxford: Blackwell Science.

Gossop, M., Stewart, D., Browne, N., & Marsden, J. (2002). Factors associated with abstinence, lapse or relapse to heroin use after residential treatment: Protective effect of coping responses. *Addiction*, 97(10), 1259–1267. https://doi.org/10.1046/j.1360-0443.2002.00227.x

Greene, D. (2021). Revisiting 12-step approaches: An evidence-based perspective, in M. Meil, & A. Mills (Eds.), *Addictions – Diagnosis and treatment*. IntechOpen. https://doi.org/10.5772/intechopen.95985

Heather, N. (1998). Using brief opportunities for change in medical settings, in W. Miller & N. Heather (Eds.), *Treating addictive behaviors*. New York: Plenum.

Heather, N., & Kaner, E. (2001). Brief Interventions: An opportunity for reducing excessive drinking. Paper presented to *Working Group: Health Systems and Alcohol at Ministerial Conference on Young People and Alcohol*, Stockholm, Sweden, 19–21 February 2001.

Heather, N., Whitton, B., & Robertson, I. (1986). Evaluation of a self-help manual for media-recruited problem drinkers: Six-month follow-up results. *The British Journal of Clinical Psychology*, 25(Pt 1), 19–34. https://doi.org/10.1111/j.2044-8260.1986.tb00667.x

Henry-Edwards, S., Humeniuk, R., Ali, R., Monteiro, M., & Poznyak. V. (2003). *Brief intervention for substance use: A manual for use in primary care.* Geneva: World Health Organization.

Howes, S., Hartmann-Boyce, J., Livingstone-Banks, J., Hong, B., & Lindson, N. (2020). Antidepressants for smoking cessation. *The Cochrane Database of Systematic Reviews*, 4(4), CD000031. https://doi. org/10.1002/14651858.CD000031.pub5

Humeniuk, R., Ali, R., Babor, T. F., Farrell, M., Formigoni, M. L., Jittiwutikarn, J., de Lacerda, R. B., Ling, W., Marsden, J., Monteiro, M., Nhiwatiwa, S., Pal, H., Poznyak, V., & Simon, S. (2008). Validation of the alcohol, smoking and substance involvement screening test (ASSIST). *Addiction*, 103(6), 1039–1047. https://doi.org/10.1111/j. 1360-0443.2007.02114.x

Humeniuk, R., Henry-Edwards, S., Ali, R., Poznyak, V., Monteiro, V., & Maristela G. (2012). *Brief intervention. The ASSIST-linked brief intervention for hazardous and harmful substance use manual for use in primary care.* Geneva: World Health Organization.

Kaner, E. F., Beyer, F. R., Muirhead, C., Campbell, F., Pienaar, E. D., Bertholet, N., Daeppen, J. B., Saunders, J. B., & Burnand, B. (2018). Effectiveness of brief alcohol interventions in primary care populations. *The Cochrane Database of Systematic Reviews*, 2(2), CD004148. https://doi.org/10.1002/14651858.CD004148.pub4

Katims, J. J., Ng, L. K. Y., & Lowinson, J. H. (1992).Acupuncture and transcutaneous electrical nerve stimulation: Afferent nerve stimulation (ANS), in K. Lowinson, P. Ruiz, R. B. Millman & J. G. Langrod (Eds.), *Treatment of addiction in substance abuse: A comprehensive textbook* (2nd ed.). Baltimore: Williams and Wilkins, pp 574–83.

Kreek, M. J., & Vocci, F. J. (2002). History and current status of opioid maintenance treatments: Blending conference session. *Journal of Substance Abuse Treatment*, 23(2), 93–105. https://doi.org/10.1016/ s0740-5472(02)00259-3

Laudet, A. B., Magura, S., Cleland, C. M., Vogel, H. S., Knight, E. L., & Rosenblum, A. (2004). The effect of 12-step based fellowship participation on abstinence among dually diagnosed persons: A two-year longitudinal study. *Journal of Psychoactive Drugs*, 36(2), 207–216.

Lilienfeld, S.O., & Arkowitz, H. (2011). Facts & fictions in mental health: Does alcoholics anonymous work? *SA Mind*, 22(1), 64.

Marissen, M. A., Franken, I. H., Blanken, P., van den Brink, W., & Hendriks, V. M. (2007). Cue exposure therapy for the treatment of opiate addiction: Results of a randomized controlled clinical trial. *Psychotherapy and Psychosomatics*, 76(2), 97–105. https://doi. org/10.1159/000097968

McDonald, L., & Rassool, G. Hussein (1997). Complementary therapies in addiction nursing practice, in G. Hussein Rassool & M. Gafoor (Eds.), *Addiction nursing: Perspectives on professional and clinical practice.* Cheltenham: Nelson Thornes.

McLellan, A. T., Wood, G. E., Metzger, D. S., McKay, J., & Altermanv, A. I. (1997). Evaluating the effectiveness of addiction treatments:

Reasonable expectations, appropriate comparisons, in J. A. Egerton, D. M. Fox & A. I. Leshner (Eds.), *Treating drug abusers effectively.* Oxford: Blackwell Publications.

Miller, W. R., & Rollnick, S. (2013). *Motivational interviewing: Helping people change.* New York: Guilford Press.

Miller, W. R., & Walker, D. D. (1997) Should there be aromatherapy for addiction? *Addiction,* 92(4), 486–487.

Moyers, T., & Hester R. K. (1999). *Textbook of substance abuse treatment.* Washington DC: American Psychiatric Press, pp. 45–65.

National Institute for Health and Clinical Excellence (NICE). (2011). *Alcohol-use disorders: Diagnosis, assessment and management of harmful drinking and alcohol dependence.* NICE clinical guidelines, no. 115. Leicester, UK: British Psychological Society, www.nice.org.uk/guidance/CG115

National Institute for Health and Clinical Excellence. NICE. (2007a). *Drug misuse in over 16s: Psychosocial interventions.* Clinical guideline 25. London: National Institute for Health and Clinical Excellence.

National Institute for Health and Clinical Excellence. NICE. (2007b). *Drug misuse: Psychosocial interventions.* NICE clinical guideline 51. London: National Institute for Health and Clinical Excellence.

National Institute for Health and Clinical Excellence. NICE. (2010). *Alcohol-use disorders: Diagnosis and clinical management of alcohol-related physical complications.* Clinical guideline 100. London: NICE.

National Institute on Drug Abuse (NIDA). (2020). *Contingency Management Interventions/Motivational Incentives (Alcohol, Stimulants, Opioids, Marijuana, Nicotine).* https://nida.nih.gov/publications/principles-drug-addiction-treatment-research-based-guide-third-edition/evidence-based-approaches-to-drug-addiction-treatment/behavioral-therapies/contingency-management-interventions-motivational-incentives on 2022, September 29, (accessed 18 January 2024).

National Institute on Drug Abuse (NIDA). (2023). *Treatment and recovery.* https://nida.nih.gov/publications/drugs-brains-behavior-science-addiction/treatment-recovery, (accessed 16 January 2024).

NTA. (2006).*Treating drug misuse problems: Evidence of effectiveness.* London: National Treatment Agency.

O'Brien, C. P., & McKay J. (2007). Psychopharmacological treatments for substance use disorders, in Peter E. Nathan, & Jack M. Gorman (Eds.), *A guide to treatments that work* (3rd ed.). Oxford Academic. https://doi.org/10.1093/med:psych/9780195304145.003.0005, (accessed 17 Jan. 2024).

Pharmaceutical Press (2013). *Joint formulary committee.* London, UK: British National Formulary.

Public Health England. (2021). *Guidance part 4: Supporting opioid detoxification.* https://www.gov.uk/government/publications/opioid-substitution-treatment-guide-for-keyworkers/part-4-supporting-opioid-detoxification, (accessed 1 March 2024).

Raistrick, D., Heather, N., & Godfrey, C. (2003). *Review of the effectiveness of treatment for alcohol problems.* London: National Treatment Agency for Substance Misuse.

Rassool, G. Hussein (Ed.). (2001). *Dual diagnosis: Substance misuse and psychiatric disorders.* Oxford: Blackwell Science.

Rassool, G. Hussein (Ed.). (2006). *Dual diagnosis nursing.* Oxford: Blackwell Publications.

Rassool, G. Hussein (2018).*Alcohol and drug misuse. A guide for health and social professionals* (2nd ed.). Oxford: Routledge.

Rassool, G. Hussein (2025). *Alcohol and drug misuse. A guide for health and social care professionals* (3rd ed.). Oxford: Routledge.

Rollnick, S., & Miller, W. R. (1995). What is motivational interviewing? *Behavioural and Cognitive Psychotherapy*, 23(4), 325–334. https://doi.org/10.1017/S135246580001643X

Sarkar, S., Pakhre, A., Murthy, P., & Bhuyan, D. (2020). Brief interventions for substance use disorders. *Indian Journal of Psychiatry*, 62(Suppl 2), S290–S298.https://doi.org/10.4103/psychiatry.IndianJPsychiatry_778_19

Schwenker, R., Dietrich, C. E., Hirpa, S., Nothacker, M., Smedslund, G., Frese, T., & Unverzagt, S. (2023). Motivational interviewing for substance use reduction. *Cochrane Database of Systematic Reviews*, 2023(12), Art. No. CD008063. https://doi.org/10.1002/14651858.CD008063.pub3

Sharma, A., Das, K., Sharma, S., & Ghosh, A. (2022). Effectiveness of 'relapse prevention therapy' on high-risk situations for alcohol use among alcohol dependents. *Nursing & Midwifery Research Journal*, 18(1), 5–12. https://doi.org/10.1177/0974150X211057957

Sing, D., & Saadabadi, A. (2023). *Naltrexone, in StatPearls [Internet].* Treasure Island (FL): StatPearls Publishing. https://www.ncbi.nlm.nih.gov/books/NBK534811/, (accessed 17 January 2024).

Sorensen, J. L., & Copeland, A. L. (2000). Drug abuse treatment as an HIV prevention strategy: A review. *Drug and Alcohol Dependence*, 59(1), 17–31. https://doi.org/10.1016/s0376-8716(99)00104-0

Spray, J. R., & Jones, S. M. (1995). The use of acupuncture in drug addiction treatment, *News Briefs.* http://www.ndsn.org/sept95/guest.html, (accessed 18 January 2024).

Stuyt, E. B., & Voyles, C. A. (2016). The National Acupuncture Detoxification Association protocol, auricular acupuncture to support clients with substance abuse and behavioral health disorders: Current perspectives. *Substance Abuse and Rehabilitation*, 7, 169–180.

Substance Abuse and Mental Health Services Administration (SAMSHA). (2021). *Treatment for stimulant use disorders.* Treatment Improvement Protocol (TIP) Series 33. SAMHSA Publication No. PEP21-02-01-004. Rockville, MD: Substance Abuse and Mental Health Services Administration.

Substance Abuse and Mental Health Services Administration. (SAMHSA). (2020). *Treatment of stimulant use disorders.* SAMHSA Publication No. PEP20-06-01-001. Rockville, MD: Substance Abuse and Mental Health Services Administration.

Teoh Bing Fei, J., Yee, A., Habil, M. H., & Danaee, M. (2016). Effectiveness of methadone maintenance therapy and improvement in quality of life following a decade of implementation. *Journal of Substance Abuse Treatment*, 69(2016), 50–56. https://doi.org/10.1016/j.jsat.2016.07.006

Thornton, P. (2023). *Naltrexone*. https://www.drugs.com/naltrexone.html, (accessed 17 January 2024).

Urits, I., Patel, A., Zusman, R., Virgen, C. G., Mousa, M., Berger, A. A., Kassem, H., Jung, J. W., Hasoon, J., Kaye, A. D., & Viswanath, O. (2020). A comprehensive update of lofexidine for the management of opioid withdrawal symptoms. *Psychopharmacology Bulletin*, 50(3), 76–96.

Velleman, R. (2011).*Counselling for alcohol problems* (3rd ed.).London: Sage Publications.

Wang, M. Y., Tsai, P. S., Lee, P. H., Chang, W. Y., & Yang, C. M. (2008). The efficacy of reflexology: Systematic review. *Journal of Advanced Nursing*, 62(5), 512–520. https://doi.org/10.1111/j.1365-2648.2008. 04606.x

WHO ASSIST Working Group. (2002). The alcohol, smoking and substance involvement screening test (ASSIST): Development, reliability and feasibility. *Addiction*, 97(9), 1183–1194.

Woody, G. E. (2003). Research findings on psychotherapy of addictive disorders. *American Journal on Addictions*, 12(Suppl. 2), S19–S26.

World Health Organization (WHO). (2009). *Clinical guidelines for withdrawal management and treatment of drug dependence in closed settings*. Geneva: World Health Organization.

5 Faith-based solutions for addiction prevention in public health

Introduction

The public health challenges associated with addiction are widespread, affecting societies globally and transcending geographical, cultural, and socio-economic boundaries. Faith-based interventions, particularly those rooted in the Islāmic faith, are being explored as preventive approaches to address addiction. Islāmic traditions emphasise holistic health, balanced lifestyles, and self-discipline, offering a unique perspective on addiction prevention. Drawing from the Qur'ân, the *hadīth*, and Islāmic jurisprudence, there is guidance on health, discipline, and avoiding harmful behaviours like alcohol and gambling. These principles contribute to a comprehensive approach to tackling addiction, recognising its multifaceted nature and the importance of spiritual dimensions in public health interventions. International efforts aim to address the supply, demand, and harm related to psychoactive substances and behavioural addictions. The historical "War on alcohol and gambling," dating back over 1400 centuries, draws parallels with the contemporary "War on drugs." Philips (2008) stresses that legislation alone cannot resolve addiction-related issues; rather, effective enforcement requires collective faith within the population. Integrating Islāmic faith-based approaches into addiction prevention in Muslim communities necessitates a comprehensive strategy.

The Islāmic approach to addiction prevention is rooted in a holistic understanding of human nature, combining spiritual guidance, education, community support, personal responsibility, promotion of alternative lifestyles, and a compassionate approach to rehabilitation. It seeks to integrate the profound teachings of Islām with evidence-based practices to create a comprehensive approach to addressing addiction within the framework of public health initiatives The chapter aims to examine prevention and public health through an Islāmic lens, specifically focusing on the Islāmic response to addiction.

DOI: 10.4324/9781032669212-5

Prevention and public health

Health and social care professionals play a crucial role in addressing addiction-related behaviours through health education, prevention, and harm reduction strategies. Public health efforts operate on three levels: primary, secondary, and tertiary prevention.

- At the primary prevention level, the focus is on preventing the onset of addiction within the broader population or specific high-risk groups. This involves implementing public awareness campaigns, provision of health information, educational initiatives, and community interventions to promote healthy behaviours and discourage substance use. The focus of primary prevention should be targeted not only to the non-using population but also to experimental, recreational, and dependent users.
- Moving to secondary prevention, the emphasis shifts to early recognition and intervention for individuals at a higher risk of developing addiction. It focuses on reducing and limiting further health and social harms done by the alcohol and drug use. Strategies at this level include screening programmes, brief interventions, and outreach efforts designed to identify and address substance use issues in their early stages, preventing the escalation of problems. By targeting individuals with identifiable risk factors, secondary prevention seeks to minimise the impact of addiction and improve outcomes through timely and targeted interventions. Those with high-risk behaviours include binge drinkers, pregnant women, youth offenders, injecting drug users, and prisoners. The harm reduction approach, often integrated into secondary preventive strategies, has found extensive application in the addiction field as a response to the threat posed by blood-borne viruses like HIV and hepatitis infections.
- Tertiary prevention addresses individuals already involved in addictive behaviours, focusing on minimising associated negative consequences. It encompasses treatment programmes, rehabilitation, support groups, and harm reduction initiatives with the goal of restoring optimal functioning and preventing relapse. This level involves engagement with residential and community facilities, often managed by specialised addiction services. Unlike primary and secondary prevention, tertiary prevention directly addresses the disease through treatment, reflecting the complexity of addiction and the necessity for tailored interventions across various stages.

Overall, these prevention strategies involve proactive measures to promote healthy behaviours, identify early signs of addiction, and mitigate risks associated with alcohol and substance use disorder, ultimately improving public health outcomes.

Harm-reduction approach

There is a growing consensus recognising that some individuals may not be ready to abstain from alcohol or drug use entirely but could still benefit from intervention. Global policies are shifting towards minimising negative consequences of drug use rather than solely emphasising abstinence, endorsed by WHO, UNODC, and UNAIDS (2012). This approach aims to prevent and alleviate problems associated with substance use, representing a significant policy and strategy change in addressing addiction. Additionally, the harm reduction approach, integrated into secondary prevention, plays a vital role in combating blood-borne viruses like HIV and hepatitis in addiction management.

Harm reduction is referred to as "policies and programmes aimed primarily at reducing the health, social and economic costs of psychotropic drugs without necessarily reducing drug consumption" (Wodak, 2009, p. 343). Another alternative definition is that Harm reduction "refers to policies, programmes and practices that aim to minimise the negative health, social and legal impacts associated with drug use, drug policies and drug laws" (Harm Reduction International). This means that harm reduction involves policies and programmes aiming to minimise the health, social, and economic costs associated with psychotropic drug use without mandating complete abstinence. The global focus on addressing drug-related harm extends to broader social and legal impacts, emphasising a comprehensive strategy to tackle the complexities surrounding drug-related issues. There has been a significant rise in the adoption of harm reduction interventions worldwide, attributed to the establishment of new needle and syringe programmes (NSPs), official sanctioning of drug consumption rooms (DCRs), take-home and peer-distribution models, and opioid agonist therapy (OAT) (Harm Reduction International, 2022). Harm reduction packages for drug use encompass a diverse set of strategies aimed at minimising the negative consequences associated with drug addiction. These include providing sterile needles, drug testing services, supervised consumption facilities, OAT, education and outreach programmes, naloxone distribution, psychotherapy or counselling, legal reforms, housing support, and peer support initiatives. The overarching goal is to reduce harm without mandating immediate abstinence, and these strategies address health risks, social factors, and the overall well-being of individuals involved in drug use.

Decades of research have consistently demonstrated the substantial individual and public health benefits associated with certain harm reduction strategies (Puzhko et al., 2022). These measures have proven effective in preventing deaths from overdoses and reducing the transmission of infectious diseases among individuals who use drugs and the broader community (Coye et al., 2021) Additionally, some harm reduction interventions have been successful in decreasing emergency department visits and lowering healthcare costs (Nassau et al., 2022, Surratt et al., 2020).

The evolving approach to alcohol misuse focuses on reducing the risk of individuals engaging in harmful drinking behaviours and moderating adverse outcomes associated with such misuse. Moderate drinking, also known as controlled drinking, is viewed as a tool to prevent potential harm associated with alcohol consumption. Rather than advocating for abstinence or resorting to shaming, moderation programmes aim to motivate individuals to reduce or quit alcohol use by allowing them to reflect on their behaviour and establish their own strategies. These programmes are designed to address alcohol misuse from a different perspective, encouraging individuals to set personal drinking limits. Research suggests that focusing on moderation can prompt individuals to seek help before their alcohol use escalates into a more serious problem (Harvard, 2022). This approach is particularly suitable for individuals who have not yet developed an alcohol use disorder. For others, moderate drinking may help prevent further harm, such as drunk driving, risky sexual activities, violence, or other potential alcohol-related problems (Marlatt & Witkiewitz, 2002).

Harm reduction strategies in alcohol consumption encompass practical measures to minimise negative consequences associated with drinking. These include specialised glassware designed to break harmlessly during pub fights, promoting safe transportation through programmes like the "Nez Rouge" ("Red Nose") programme for individuals who have consumed excessive alcohol at events or licensed establishments, the availability of low-alcohol beverages, and controlled drinking programmes tailored for chaotic alcohol users (Single & Storm, 1985; Single, 1996). Other strategies may include responsible alcohol service training, designated driver programmes, education campaigns, brief interventions, restrictions on high-strength alcohol availability, safe drinking spaces, community engagement, treatment services, and early intervention programmes. The goals are to promote responsible drinking behaviours, raise awareness, and provide support without mandating complete abstinence. These strategies address various aspects of alcohol consumption to reduce harm and encourage safer practices. Harm reduction approaches in the context of alcohol now extend beyond a generalised approach and instead focus on specific risk behaviours, target groups, and drinking contexts, as highlighted by Rassool (2018, p. 348).

Recent studies challenge the notion that moderate alcohol consumption provides protective health benefits, such as reducing the risk of heart disease, a claim supported by past research (CDC, 2022). Contrary to earlier findings, current studies suggest that the positive health outcomes associated with moderate drinking may not be conclusively linked to alcohol consumption. The difficulty arises from the inability to determine whether the observed health improvements among moderate drinkers result from alcohol intake itself or stem from other factors, such as distinct behaviours or genetic variations, which may differ between moderate drinkers and non-drinkers (CDC, 2022). The ambiguity in these recent findings raises questions about the previously assumed health advantages of moderate alcohol consumption.

Prevention and public health in addiction: An Islāmic perspective

The policy of the first Islāmic state incorporated prevention and public health, suggesting that practices such as good hygiene, nutrition, disease prevention, and infectious disease control, as revealed through prophetic tradition, align with modern public health principles. These practices, grounded in Islām, emphasise the religion's holistic approach to life, encompassing public health. Over 1,440 years ago, Islām advocated for fundamental public health principles that are still recognised today. The Qur'ân emphasises prevention, known as *wiqaya*, against negative actions (*wiqayat min al sayi'at*) (Kasule, 2016), such as the alcohol, gambling or games of chance. In guiding individuals on health and virtue, both the Qur'ân and the Sunnah provide teachings that emphasise the importance of protecting one's health. Overall, Islām places significant emphasis on health and prevention, reflecting principles that remain relevant in contemporary public health practices. Allāh mentions in the Qur'ân:

وَلْتَكُن مِّنكُمْ أُمَّةٌ يَدْعُونَ إِلَى ٱلْخَيْرِ وَيَأْمُرُونَ بِٱلْمَعْرُوفِ وَيَنْهَوْنَ عَنِ ٱلْمُنكَرِ ۚ وَأُوْلَٰئِكَ هُمُ ٱلْمُفْلِحُونَ

And let there be [arising] from you a nation inviting to [all that is] good; enjoining what is right and forbidding what is wrong, and those will be the successful.

(Ali-'Imran 3: 104, interpretation of the meaning)

This verse emphasises the importance of fostering a community committed to promoting good, upholds righteousness and actions and discourages immoral behaviour. It reflects the Islāmic principle of enjoining good and forbidding evil as a means to cultivate a virtuous and just community. On the authority of Abu Sa'eed al-Khudree (may Allāh be pleased with him) who said: I heard the Messenger of Allāh (ﷺ) said,

Whosoever of you sees an evil, let him change it with his hand; and if he is not able to do so, then [let him change it] with his tongue; and if he is not able to do so, then with his heart – and that is the weakest of faith.

(Muslim)

The teachings of Islām are designed to bring benefit (*maslahah*) to individuals and communities while preventing harm (*mafsadah*). It is evident that these teachings have the overarching goal of preserving five fundamental aspects: human life, intellect, property, family, and religion (Al-Raysuni, 2011). For example, the prohibition of alcohol consumption and gambling, all aim to achieve preserving those five objectives of the *Shar'iah*. The Qur'ân and *hadīths* provide numerous directives on maintaining health at the community, family, and individual levels, making the prevention of addiction and gambling a paramount concern. Ignoring the role of Islām in a community, as suggested by Simpson (2005), is viewed as inviting failure for any public health programme, including undertakings such as polio eradication, HIV prevention, or tobacco control. The teachings of Islām are considered integral to the success and effectiveness of public health initiatives, reinforcing the importance of incorporating Islāmic principles into health programmes for optimal community well-being.

Islām's approach to public health aligns with an "upstream approach," emphasising primary prevention over treatment by addressing the root causes of disease and disability (Rassool, 2021). This concept, illustrated by the analogy of people drowning in a river, emphasises that rescue efforts alone are insufficient; instead, the focus should be on understanding why individuals are falling into the river in the first place. In the context of Islām, this approach reflects the religion's emphasis on preventive measures and addressing fundamental causes to enhance the overall well-being of individuals and communities. Islām's proactive stance towards public health aligns with the principles of upstream prevention, recognising the importance of addressing issues at their source for lasting positive outcomes. One of the principles of Islāmic jurisprudence known as *Sadd adh-dhara'i* provides a good example of the importance of prevention in Islām. As a doctrine of Islāmic jurisprudence, it refers to blocking the means to evil. Kamali (2006) stated:

> The whole concept of *Sadd al-dhara'i* is founded in the idea of preventing an evil before it actually materialises. It is therefore not always necessary that the result should actually take place. It is rather the objective expectation that a means is likely to lead to an evil result that renders the means in question unlawful even without the realisation of the expected result.
>
> (p. 268)

Sadd al-dhara'i in Islām emphasises a proactive approach to safeguarding against harm before it becomes a reality. This principle highlights the importance of avoiding actions that may lead to harm, reflecting an ethical and moral stance in Islāmic legal philosophy.

Islāmic response to the addiction problem

During the early formative period of *Fiqh* (Islāmic jurisprudence), which spans the first and second centuries of the Hijra (7th to 8th centuries CE), early Islāmic jurists did not record specific rulings on drug use for several reasons. As Safian (2013) notes, during this period, drugs were primarily known for their beneficial effects, and their lawful usage was widely accepted. At the time, the use of various substances was often associated with medicinal or therapeutic purposes. As time progressed, with the spread and diversification of psychoactive substances such as opium, hashish, and khat and the emergence of societal issues related to use, Islāmic jurists began to address these concerns. This prompted the jurists to revisit and adapt legal principles. This is in line with the dynamic nature of *Fiqh*, which allows for the adaptation of legal rulings to address new and emerging issues faced by the Muslim community.

Islāmic teachings explicitly prohibit the consumption of intoxicants and gambling, as explicitly stated in the Qur'ân and *hadīths*. This prohibition forms the basis of a preventive approach to addiction within the Islāmic framework, emphasising proactive avoidance of substances and activities that may lead to dependence or intoxication. By prohibiting intoxicants and gambling, Islām aims to safeguard individuals' physical, mental, and spiritual well-being, viewing addiction not only as a personal failing but also as a deviation from the righteous path. This preventive strategy recognises the detrimental effects of such substances on individuals and society, aligning with broader Islāmic principles of promoting virtue and righteousness. It highlights the importance of personal responsibility and self-discipline, encouraging individuals to make choices that preserve their well-being and contribute to the overall welfare of the community. The holistic nature of Islāmic teachings addresses not only the physical aspects of addiction but also its spiritual and societal dimensions.

The landscape of addressing addiction from an Islāmic perspective has been transformed by the issues of HIV and blood-borne infections. Despite previous perceptions of protection due to religious and cultural norms, Muslim countries globally are experiencing a rapidly increasing threat of HIV/AIDS. This rise is attributed to changes in lifestyles and behaviours influenced by acculturation, unprotected sexual intercourse, LGBT+ issues, sex work, and shared injection equipment. Islām plays a crucial role in addressing the HIV/AIDS epidemic, primarily through prevention efforts. In the Middle East and North Africa (MENA) region, the adoption of harm reduction approaches remains limited, with only nine out of 19 nations implementing any form of harm reduction program (Harm Reduction International, 2020). Notably, Bahrain and Kuwait, located in this region, discontinued OAT programmes recently, while Egypt has initiated OAT programmes (Harm Reduction International,

2023). The overall reluctance to embrace harm reduction measures in MENA, especially in the Middle East, emphasises a significant gap in addressing substance use disorder and HIV prevention challenges in these countries.

However, the challenge of HIV/AIDS prevention in Muslim countries is complicated by various factors, including the prevalent social stigma surrounding addiction. Some Muslims lack awareness that HIV can be transmitted through means other than immoral sexual behaviours. They may be unaware of mother-to-child transmission or the risk of contamination through blood, needles, or from an infected spouse. Reasons for the spread of HIV in Muslim countries are speculative, considering Islām's emphasis on faithful behaviour and prohibition of extramarital sex, adultery, and intoxicants. However, risky behaviours such alcohol and drug use and commercial sex exist in Muslim countries, contributing to HIV transmission. Western acculturation, ignorance, and misinformation further complicate the issue. Given the spread of psychoactive substances and the prevalence of HIV and blood-borne infections in Muslim communities, it becomes imperative to consider strategies, including a harm reduction approach. This perspective may initially be considered unconventional in Islāmic contexts due to the religious prohibition of intoxicants and the emphasis on moral conduct. However, contemplating a harm reduction approach is necessary to address the dual challenges of addiction and HIV transmission.

Thinking the unthinkable: Harm reduction approach from an Islāmic perspective

Harm reduction approaches aim to minimise the negative consequences of addictive and injecting behaviours, particularly in controlling the HIV pandemic. Evidence suggests success with such strategies in several Muslim-majority countries. Notably, the Islāmic Republic of Iran (Cook, 2010; Nissaramanesh et al., 2005), Malaysia (Bin Shaikh Mohd Salleh & Kamarulzaman, 2016; Reid & Kamarulzaman, 2007), and Indonesia (Mesquita et al., 2007) have implemented harm reduction measures, including needle exchange programmes and opioid substitution therapy. Iran notably stands out as the only country in the region significantly expanding both needle exchange programmes and opioid substitution therapy (Cook, 2010). These initiatives have effectively reduced HIV transmission and mitigated substance use-related harms in these Islāmic countries. Evaluations of harm reduction programmes in Malaysia have shown them to be cost-effective, averting approximately 12,000 new HIV infections (Bin Shaikh Mohd Salleh & Kamarulzaman, 2016). While some Muslim countries have rejected harm reduction approaches for intravenous drug use-driven HIV epidemics, others have introduced needle and syringe programmes (NSPs operating through both fixed and mobile units. Provision of opioid substitution therapy has been reported in Iran, Lebanon, Morocco, Egypt, and the UAE.

In many Islāmic countries, there is resistance to embracing harm reduction strategies despite the prevalence of substance use and HIV epidemics linked to intravenous drug use. Religious and political leaders typically oppose measures like needle distribution, condom distribution, and opioid substitution therapy, fearing endorsement of drug use and illicit sexual relations (Reid & Kamarulzaman, 2007). Critics argue that harm reduction contradicts Islāmic rules and values, making it unacceptable for HIV prevention (Madani et al., 2004). Instead, they advocate for strengthening Islāmic and health education, promoting adherence to Islāmic principles prohibiting adultery, homosexuality, and drug use, and advocating for safe sex within legal marriage as more suitable strategies for preventing HIV infection (Madani et al., 2004). Opioid substitution therapy is viewed as deterring the goal of a drug-free society. This clash between public health approaches and religious beliefs highlights the need to find solutions that effectively address HIV while respecting cultural and religious frameworks. Discussions surrounding harm reduction in Islāmic countries are influenced by complex interplays of religious, cultural, and political factors.

In Islāmic countries, proponents of harm reduction strategies to combat drug-related HIV epidemics ground their arguments in the Islāmic principles of "*Maqâsid Ash-Shar'iah.*" *Maqâsid Ash-Shar'iah*, the Higher objectives or goals of Islāmic law, plays a significant role in shaping the perspective on harm reduction within the context of Islāmic principles. The primary objectives of *Maqâsid Ash-Shari'ah* include the preservation and protection of essential values, known as the five Maqâsid: faith, life, intellect, progeny, and wealth. Understanding how harm reduction aligns with these objectives is crucial for evaluating its permissibility within an Islāmic framework. According to Kamarulzaman and Saifuddeen (2010), harm reduction programmes are deemed permissible within Islāmic principles and offer a practical solution to preventing greater societal damage if unaddressed. The authors highlight the Islāmic principle that prohibits causing harm to oneself or others, supporting the "lesser of the two evils" principle.

In the context of opiate substitution treatment and needle exchange programmes or the gamut of harm reduction, several provisions within *Shar'iah*, the Islāmic legal framework, can be invoked. The Islāmic legal maxim "*La dharar wa la dhirar,*" captures the principle that harm must be removed or avoided, serving as a fundamental concept within the broader framework of *Qawā'id al-Fiqhiyyah*, or legal maxims in Islāmic jurisprudence. This maxim, meaning "No harm shall be inflicted or reciprocated," underlines the preventive nature of Islāmic ethics, encouraging actions that prioritise the well-being of individuals and society. Embracing an ethical foundation rooted in compassion and justice, the maxim allows for adaptability to changing circumstances while maintaining a core focus on harm prevention. In the case of alcohol and drug addiction, and HIV/AIDS, which bring about significant harm to individuals and their families in terms of life and health, Islāmic principles emphasise the mitigation of harm to the greatest extent possible. Islāmic jurisprudence aligns with the idea that "a lesser harm may be tolerated in order to eliminate a greater harm." This principle recognises the necessity of adopting measures such as opiate substitution treatment and needle exchange programmes to address the serious consequences of drug addiction and the spread of HIV/AIDS. By endorsing harm reduction strategies, Islāmic principles underline the ethical imperative to prioritise public health and well-being, allowing for the acceptance of certain interventions that may be considered a lesser harm in order to prevent more significant and widespread harm within society.

The principle "*Al-dharurat tuhibul mahzurat,*" which translates to "Necessities override prohibitions," holds significance in the context of harm reduction within Islāmic jurisprudence. This principle acknowledges that, in cases of great necessity, actions that are normally prohibited may become permissible to address pressing needs.

فَمَنِ ٱضْطُرَّ غَيْرَ بَاغٍ وَلَا عَادٍ فَلَا إِثْمَ عَلَيْهِ

But whoever is forced [by necessity], neither desiring [it] nor transgressing [its limit], there is no sin upon him.
(Al-Baqarah 2:173, interpretation of the meaning)

وَمَا جَعَلَ عَلَيْكُمْ فِى ٱلدِّينِ مِنْ حَرَجٍ

...and He has not placed upon you in the religion any difficulty.
(Al-Hajj 22:78, interpretation of the meaning)

فَصَّلَ لَكُم مَّا حَرَّمَ عَلَيْكُمْ إِلَّا مَا ٱضْطُرِرْتُمْ

...while He has explained in detail to you what He has forbidden you, excepting that to which you are compelled.
(Al-An'am 6:119, interpretation of the meaning)

The Qur'ânic verses underline this principle. The verses recognise the permissibility of consuming forbidden (*harām*) substances in cases of dire necessity. The general meaning of the verse is that Allāh has permitted certain exemptions in specific situations, particularly when individuals are compelled by extreme circumstances and have no other option but to consume what is normally prohibited. The Islāmic principle "Necessities overrule prohibitions" allows for exemptions in extreme circumstances where individuals have no choice but to consume what is normally prohibited. This pragmatic approach aligns with the broader Islāmic values of compassion, justice, and the preservation of life and well-being. It acknowledges that certain prohibitions may be overridden to address pressing needs or avert greater harm, emphasising the adaptability of Islāmic law to real-world challenges. In essence, the principle highlights the priority to choose the lesser of two evils to prevent more severe consequences. This pragmatic approach in Islāmic jurisprudence underlines a commitment to prioritise the well-being and safety of individuals and society, even if it requires temporarily setting aside certain prohibitions for the greater good.

The "lesser of two evils" principle in Islāmic law, known as "*Istislah*" or "choosing the lesser harm," is a juristic concept that allows for the permissibility of an action that may otherwise be considered unlawful or discouraged, if it prevents a greater harm or evil. This principle is derived from the broader Islāmic legal framework and ethical considerations, seeking to balance the preservation of fundamental values and the avoidance of harm. Shaykh Al-Islām Ibn Taymiyyah (may Allāh have mercy upon him) stated, "Benefits should be realised and perfected, and evils should be eliminated and reduced; in case of a clash, realising the greater of two benefits or enduring the lesser of two evils is the prescribed action in this regard." This means that the emphasis is on the maximisation of benefits and minimisation of harms. It aligns with the ethical principle of realising greater benefits or enduring lesser evils. However, evils and harms,. from addiction, must be eliminated or avoided as long as this is possible, based on the well-known Fiqh principles: "Harm must be eliminated," and, "There should be neither harm nor reciprocal harm." It was related to the authority of Abu Sa'id Sa'd bin Malik bin Sinan al-Khudri (may Allāh have mercy upon him) that the Messenger of Allāh (ﷺ) said: "There should be neither harming nor reciprocating harm" (Ibn Majah, Al-Daraqutni). However, if both evils cannot be eliminated or avoided and there is no other way but to choose one of two evils, then one should opt for the lesser of the two.

The principle "*Dafu al-dharar wa jalbul manfaat*," which translates to "Harm must be treated, and benefits must be brought forth," focuses on the importance of addressing harm and promoting benefits within Islāmic jurisprudence. Applied to harm reduction, this principle emphasises mitigating harm, particularly concerning behaviours or conditions detrimental to individuals and society. This principle aligns with the idea that efforts should focus on treating or minimising harm caused by issues like gambling, alcohol and drug addiction or disease spread, while also striving for positive outcomes. It supports implementing measures such as needle exchange programmes or opioid substitution therapy to reduce negative consequences of certain lifestyle behaviours, aiming not only to treat harm but also to promote overall well-being.

The maxim of the *Qawā'id al-Fiqhiyyah* "Hardship begets facility" reflects a principle in Islāmic jurisprudence that acknowledges the flexibility and adaptability of Islāmic law in the face of hardship or necessity. Known as "*Al-Mashaqqah Tajlib At-Taysir*," this principle suggests that ease or facilitation is provided in matters of religious practice or law when faced with difficulties or challenges. Applied to harm reduction, this principle implies that in situations where strict adherence to prohibitions may lead to significant harm or difficulty, flexibility and facilitation should be considered to address challenges effectively. In the realm of harm reduction, this principle aligns with the idea that pragmatic and adaptive measures should be considered to alleviate difficulties caused by issues such as drug addiction or spread of disease, prioritising the well-being of individuals and society.

When applying Islāmic jurisprudential maxims, particularly those related to harm reduction, advocates must establish a compelling case that greater harm will occur if certain measures are not taken. This requirement aligns with principles like necessity overruling prohibitions and enduring the lesser of two evils to prevent a graver one. In other words, the burden of proof lies in demonstrating that not implementing harm reduction strategies would result in more significant and undesirable consequences for individuals and society. In the context of harm reduction, advocates may need to provide evidence of potential harms associated with issues like drug addiction and the spread of infections such as HIV/ AIDS through intravenous drug use. This evidence could include data on prevalence rates, public health impacts, and potential societal repercussions. By establishing a clear link between the current situation and potential harm, proponents can make a case for the necessity of harm reduction measures.

Ummah and *Imam* response to addiction

Harm reduction from an Islāmic perspective involves a multifaceted approach incorporating psychosocial, pharmacological, and spiritual interventions. Positioned within a continuum from addiction to total abstinence, the ultimate treatment goal for Muslims struggling with substance use disorder or gambling is abstinence. Strategies include promoting Islāmic values through educational programmes and media campaigns based on Qur'ânic verses and *hadīths*, strengthening family and community ties through therapy, counselling, mentorship, and community events. Addiction prevention education, integrated into Islāmic curriculum for various age groups, addresses the health and spiritual consequences of substance use, gambling, and social media misuse. Providing alternative activities such as sports and cultural programmes aims to offer positive alternatives to substance use among youth and adults. The comprehensive approach aims to establish resilient, supportive environments aligned with Islāmic principles to prevent addiction within Muslim populations.

Community leaders, particularly *Imams*, or faith-leaders, play a pivotal role in addressing social issues such as alcohol and drug use, gambling, pornography, and cyber addiction. Studies like Padela et al. (2010) highlight the involvement of *Imams* in healthcare-related roles, including promoting healthy behaviours through scripture-based messages in sermons. Imam Muhammed Asim Hussain (2018) emphasises the urgency of openly addressing issues like drug and alcohol use, crime, and domestic abuse. While *Imams* dealing with addiction represent a minority, they increasingly address these issues in Friday *khutbahs* (sermons). There is a growing recognition of the importance of community organisations collaborating with mosques and *Imams* to collectively address addiction problems, aiming for a more comprehensive and effective approach to tackling substance abuse within the community.

The following example is good practice in dealing with those with addictions. It is about the Turkish *Imam* who has brought dozens of individuals struggling with substance use disorder back from the brink (Tasci, 2021). The Turkish *Imam* Kir exemplifies effective and compassionate practices in dealing with individuals struggling with addiction. Over 15 years, *Imam* Kir, known as "baba" or father, has played a pivotal role in the recovery of dozens of former individuals with addiction in Istanbul, Turkey. His approach is characterised by an inclusive and non-judgemental attitude, stating that when individuals seek help, their religion or background is not questioned; they are first recognised as human beings deserving of mercy. Operating from the perspective that the mosque is a space embracing people from all walks of life, *Imam* Kir, with the support of the local community, provides essential services such as accommodation, meals, and tea to those in need. *Imam* Kir's unique approach involves addressing the needs of drug users with empathy, support, and inclusive care in fostering recovery and rebuilding lives affected by addiction.

Research by Mustafa et al. (2017) and Mallik et al. (2021) examines the role of *Imams* and mosques in health promotion within Western societies, particularly regarding substance use disorders (SUD) among Muslim Americans. Mallik et al. (2021) found that *Imams'* perspectives on individuals with SUD varied from focusing on sin, shame, and social disruption to emphasising acceptance and forgiveness. Stigma surrounding addiction and mental health issues in Muslim communities acts as a barrier to seeking help, necessitating education on Islāmic teachings and addiction's nature. Transformational leaders, scholars, and *Imams* can counter stigma by promoting empathy, compassion, and reducing judgement, crucial for individuals, families, and significant others affected by addiction. Culturally sensitive services and increased Muslim representation in mental health services can shift perceptions, while media and social networks can combat prejudice and stigma surrounding addiction and mental health in the Muslim community.

Conclusion

The Islāmic response to addiction incorporates primary prevention principles by promoting awareness, psychological interventions, and spiritual development. The systematic desensitisation approach aligns with Islāmic teachings, emphasising gradual change and purification of the soul. This comprehensive approach aims to address addiction at its roots, fostering a society based on spiritual well-being and adherence to ethical principles. Dealing with alcohol addiction or any form of addictive behaviours is considered both a community obligation (*Fard kifaya*) and an individual obligation ('*Ayn kifaya*) within Islāmic teachings. This signifies that the responsibility to address and combat addiction is shared by the community as a whole, but each individual also bears a personal obligation to contribute to finding solutions with the help of Allāh. In the Islāmic context, this highlights the collective and individual duty to address and mitigate the challenges posed by addiction through community support, education, and compassionate interventions.

References

Al-Raysuni, A. (2011). *Imam Al-Shatibi's theory of the higher objectives and intents of Islāmic law*. Herndon, VA: International Institute of Islāmic Thought.

Bin Shaikh Mohd Salleh, S. M. S., & Kamarulzaman, A. (2016). Implementation of an Islāmic approach to harm reduction among illicit drug users in Malaysia, in M. Kamali, Bakar, O., Batchelor, D. F., & Hashim, R. (Eds.), *Islāmic perspectives on science and technology*. Singapore: Springer. https://doi.org/10.1007/978-981-287-778-9_18

Centers for Disease Control and Prevention. (2022). *Dietary guidelines for alcohol*. https://www.cdc.gov/alcohol/fact-sheets/moderate-drinking. htm#:~:text=Although%20past%20studies%20have%20indicated% 20that%20moderate%20alcohol,who%20drink%20moderately% 20and%20people%20who%20don%E2%80%99t.%206-12, (accessed 19 January 2024).

Cook, C. (2010). *Global state of harm reduction: Key issues for broadening the response*. London: International Harm Reduction Association.

Coye, A. E., Bornstein, K. J., Bartholomew, T. S., Li, H., Wong, S., Janjua, N. Z., Tookes, H. E., & St Onge, J. E. (2021). Hospital costs of injection drug use in Florida. *Clinical Infectious Diseases: An Official Publication* of the *Infectious Diseases Society of America*, 72(3), 499–502. https://doi.org/10.1093/cid/ciaa823

Harm Reduction International. (2020). *Global state of harm reduction.* London: Harm Reduction International.

Harm Reduction International. (2022) *Global state of harm reduction 2022.* London: Harm Reduction International.

Harm Reduction International. (2023) *Global state of harm reduction: 2023 update to key data.* London: Harm Reduction International.

Harm Reduction International. *What is harm reduction?* https://hri.global/what-is-harm-reduction/, (accessed 18 January 2024).

Harvard. (2022). Alcohol: Balancing risks and benefits. https://www.hsph.harvard.edu/nutritionsource/healthy-drinks/drinks-to-consume-in-moderation/alcohol-full-story/, (accessed 19 January 2024).

Ibn Majah, Al-Daraqutni. *The forty Hadith of Imam Nawawi.* Hādīth 32. https://40hadithnawawi.com/hadith/32-no-harming-nor-reciprocating-harm/, (accessed 20 January 2024).

Ibn Taymiyya. *Majmoo' Al-Fataawa* (Saudi ed.). Cork, Ireland: Sifatu Safwa Corporation.

Imam Muhammed Asim Hussain. (2018).Cited in Jagger, D. *Imam Muhammed Asim Hussain calls on Muslim community to tackle dangerous driving and drug and gun crime.* https://www.thetelegraphandargus.co.uk/news/16406746.imam-muhammed-asim-hussain-calls-muslim-community-tackle-dangerous-driving-drug-gun-crime/, (accessed 12 January 2024).

Kamali, M. H. (2006). *Principles of Islāmic jurisprudence* (New Third Revised & Enlarged ed.). Cambridge: Islāmic Texts Society.

Kamarulzaman, A., & Saifuddeen, S. M. (2010). Islam and harm reduction. *The International Journal on Drug Policy*, 21(2), 115–118. https://doi.org/10.1016/j.drugpo.2009.11.003

Kasule, O. (2016). *A Qur'ânic approach to disease prevention and cure.* https://muslimvillage.com/2016/03/17/6872/role-of-Islām-in-disease-prevention-and-cure/, (accessed 19 January 2024).

Madani, T. A., Al-Mazrou, Y. Y., Al-Jeffri, M. H., & Al Huzaim, N. S. (2004). Epidemiology of the human immunodeficiency virus in Saudi Arabia; 18-year surveillance results and prevention from an Islāmic perspective. *BMC Infectious Diseases*, 4, 25. https://doi.org/10.1186/1471-2334-4-25

Mallik, S., Starrels, J. L., Shannon, C., Edwards, K., & Nahvi, S. (2021). "An undercover problem in the Muslim community": A qualitative study of imams' perspectives on substance use. *Journal of Substance Abuse Treatment*, 123, 108224. https://doi.org/10.1016/j.jsat.2020.108224

Marlatt, G. A. & Witkiewitz, K. (2002). Harm reduction approaches to alcohol use: Health promotion, prevention, and treatment. *Addictive Behaviors*, 27(6), 867–886.

Mesquita, F., Winsarno, I., Atmosukarto, I. I., Eka, B., Nevendorff, I,. Rahmah, A., Handoyo, P., Anastasia, P., & Angela, R. (2007). Public health the leading force of the Indonesian response to the HIV/AIDS crisis among people who inject drugs. *Harm Reduction Journal*, 4(1) 9.

Muslim. *Hadith 34, 40 Hadith an-Nawawi.* https://sunnah.com/nawawi40:34

Mustafa, Y., Baker, D., Puligari, P., Melody, T., Yeung, J., & Gao-Smith, F. (2017). The role of imams and mosques in health promotion in Western societies – A systematic review protocol. *Systematic Reviews*, 6(1), 25. https://doi.org/10.1186/s13643-016-0404-4

Nassau, T., Kolla, G., Mason, K., Hopkins, S., Tookey, P., McLean, E., Werb, D., & Scheim, A. (2022). Service utilization patterns and characteristics among clients of integrated supervised consumption sites in Toronto, Canada. *Harm Reduction Journal*, 19(1), 33. https://doi.org/10.1186/s12954-022-00610-y

Nissaramanesh, B., Trace, M., & Roberts, M. (2005). *The rise of harm reduction in the Islāmic Republic of Iran.* The Beckley Foundation Drug Policy Programme (BFDPP). http://www.akzept.org/pdf/presse_pdf/nr18/iran_paperbeckley.pdf, (accessed 20 January 2024).

Padela, A., Killawi, A., Heisler, M., Demonner, S., & Fetters M. (2010). The role of Imams in American Muslim health: Perspectives of Muslim Community Leaders in Southeast Michigan. *Journal of Religion and Health.* 50(2), 359–373. https://doi.org/10.1007/s10943-010-9428-6

Philips, A. B. (2008). *War on drugs began 14 centuries ago.* https://d1.Islāmhouse.com/data/en/ih_articles/single/en_War_on_drugs.pdf, (accessed 18 January 2024).

Puzhko, S., Eisenberg, M. J., Filion, K. B., Windle, S. B., Hébert-Losier, A., Gore, G., Paraskevopoulos, E., Martel, M. O., & Kudrina, I. (2022). Effectiveness of interventions for prevention of common infections among opioid users: A systematic review of systematic reviews. *Frontiers in Public Health*, 10, 749033. https://doi.org/10.3389/fpubh.2022.749033

Rassool, G. Hussein. (2018). *Alcohol and drug misuse. A guide for health and social care professionals* (2nd ed.). Oxford: Routledge.

Rassool, G. Hussein. (2021). *Mother of all evils: Addictive behaviours from an Islāmic perspective.* London: Islāmic Psychology Publishing (IPP) & Institute of Islāmic Psychology Research (RIIPR). Amazon/Kindle.

Reid, G. A., & Kamarulzaman, S. K. (2007). Malaysia and harm reduction: The challenges and responses. *International Journal of Drug Policy*, 18(2), 136–140.

Safian, Y. H. M. (2013).An analysis on Islāmic rules on drugs. *International Journal of Education and Research*, 1(9), 1–16.

Simpson, B.W. (2005). *The Muslim Mosaic –Islām and Public Health.* https://magazine.jhsph.edu/2005/spring/muslim_mosaic/index.html, (accessed 19 January 2024).

Single, E. (1996). Harm reduction as an alcohol-prevention strategy. *Alcohol Health and Research World*, 20(4), 239–243.

Single, E., & Storm, T. (Eds.) (1985). *Public drinking and public policy.* Toronto: Addiction Research Foundation.

Surratt, H. L., Otachi, J. K., Williams, T., Gulley, J., Lockard, A. S., & Rains, R. (2020). Motivation to change and treatment participation among syringe service program utilizers in Rural Kentucky. *The Journal of Rural Health: Official Journal of the American Rural Health Association and the National Rural Health Care Association*, 36(2), 224–233. https://doi.org/10.1111/jrh.12388

Tasci, U. N. (2021). *The Imam in Istanbul who became a 'father' to drug addicts.* https://www.trtworld.com/magazine/the-imam-in-istanbul-who-became-a-father-to-drug-addicts-44326, (accessed 20 January 2024).

WHO, UNODC, UNAIDS. (2012). *Technical guide for countries to set targets for universal access to HIV prevention, treatment and care for injecting drug users-2012 revision.* https://iris.who.int/bitstream/handle/10665/77969/9789241504379_eng.pdf?sequence=1, (accessed 19 January 2024).

Wodak, A. (2009). Harm reduction is now the mainstream global drug policy. *Addiction*, 104(3), 343–346. https://doi.org/10.1111/j.1360-0443.2008.02440.x

6 Tawbah (repentance) in Islām

Understanding the process of change

Introduction

The initial stage for a Muslim addict who is prepared to quit involves seeking repentance (*tawbah*),. From an Islāmic perspective, "repentance (*tawbah*) has to do with the relationship between the individual and Allāh, the Almighty, as they are inherent moral, psychological and spiritual factors in the process and experience of repentance" (Rassool, 2021, p. 26). In Islāmic teachings, *tawbah* is a process of turning back to Allāh, acknowledging one's mistakes, expressing sincere remorse, and making a commitment to change one's behaviour. For a Muslim struggling with addiction, this signifies a spiritual and personal initiative to seek forgiveness and divine guidance in the journey towards recovery. *Tawbah* serves as a foundational step, aligning with Islāmic principles that emphasise repentance and the opportunity for redemption. It highlights the spiritual aspect of the recovery process, linking faith with the commitment to overcoming addictive behaviours. Unlike the concept of original sin in Christian traditions, Islām does not emphasise the need for atonement or confession. At an individual level, the first step towards recovery is to sincerely repent, acknowledging mistakes and seeking forgiveness.

This chapter aims to explore the concept of *tawbah* from an Islāmic perspective and apply the transtheoretical model (TTM) of change to understand the behavioural transformation from engaging in sinful actions to the process of repentance. The focus is to provide a comprehensive understanding of how individuals, from an Islāmic standpoint, progress through the stages of behaviour change, ultimately leading to repentance as a transformative process.

Sins and transgressions

In Western Christian theology, the concept of original sin stems from Adam and Eve's disobedience in eating a forbidden fruit in the Garden of Eden. This led to the belief that everyone is born inherently sinful with a

DOI: 10.4324/9781032669212-6

predisposition to guilt, separation from God, and disobedience. This condition is seen as a result of the first human transgression and brings feelings of remorse and guilt into human lives. In contrast, Islāmic theology does not embrace the notion of original sin as found in Western Christian theology. According to Islāmic beliefs, there is no inherent sinful condition from birth. Instead, Islām emphasises the concept of *"fitrah."* Fitrah refers to the innate and natural disposition or primordial nature with which every human being is born. The essence of the *fitrah* is the natural spiritual nature of man and having a predisposition to submit to the One God and to love God, truth, and beauty. "The *fitrah* embodies the notion that humans begin life not with blank moral slates (tabula rasa) but are hardwired with an innate sense of morality and truth. The idea of *fitrah* aligns with the Islāmic understanding that humans are born with the potential for goodness and righteousness, and it is their actions and choices that determine their moral standing and ethical behaviours.

Additionally, there is a notable difference between the concept of sinning in Islām and Christianity. In Islām, there is no recognition of "sinning in the mind," and an evil thought is not considered sinful until acted upon. Overcoming and dismissing evil thoughts are seen as deserving of reward rather than punishment in Islāmic teachings. This distinction highlights the varying perspectives on the nature of human sinfulness and its consequences in the two theological traditions. The following *hādīth* echoes the statement Narrated Abu Hurayrah (may Allāh be pleased with him): The Prophet (ﷺ) said, "Allāh has forgiven my followers the evil thoughts that occur to their minds, as long as such thoughts are not put into action or uttered." And Qatada said, "If someone divorces his wife just in his mind, such an unuttered divorce has no effect" (Bukhârî (a)).

Sinning is acknowledged as inherent in human nature and is considered an obstacle to spiritual development. Recognising that human beings have flaws and weaknesses, it is these inherent imperfections that may lead individuals to engage in deviant behaviour. Basiony (2017) suggests that while complete avoidance of sin may be impossible, individuals have the capacity to exercise control over their sinful tendencies. This control can be achieved through efforts to discipline the lower self (*an-nafs al-ʾammārah*), purify thoughts and actions, engage in virtuous deeds, surround oneself with righteous companions, and engage in regular repentance. The emphasis is on self-discipline and moral purification as means to mitigate the impact of human errors and foster spiritual growth. It is reported Nawwas ibn Sam'an asked the Messenger of Allāh (ﷺ), about righteousness and sin. He said, "Righteousness is good character and sin is what gnaws at your conscience and that which you dislike for other people to become aware of" (Al-Adab Al-Mufrad (a)). Sins tend to blemish the heart and the *nafs* and induce emotional grief, sorrow, guilt, remorse, and pain for most individuals. Abu Hurayrah (may Allāh be pleased with him): narrated that the Messenger of Allāh (ﷺ), said:

> Verily, when the slave (of Allāh) commits a sin, a black spot appears on his heart. When he refrains from it, seeks forgiveness and repents, his heart is polished clean. But if he returns, it increases until it covers his entire heart. And that is the "Ran" which Allāh mentioned: "Nay, but on their hearts is the Ran which they used to earn."
>
> (Tirmidhî)

The following is the Qur'ānic and *hadīth* guidance on sins. Allāh says in the Qur'ān:

$$\text{قُلْ يَٰعِبَادِىَ ٱلَّذِينَ أَسْرَفُواْ عَلَىٰٓ أَنفُسِهِمْ لَا تَقْنَطُواْ مِن رَّحْمَةِ ٱللَّهِ ۚ إِنَّ ٱللَّهَ يَغْفِرُ ٱلذُّنُوبَ جَمِيعًا ۚ إِنَّهُۥ هُوَ ٱلْغَفُورُ ٱلرَّحِيمُ}$$

Say, "O My servants who have transgressed against themselves [by sinning], do not despair of the mercy of Allāh. Indeed, it is He who is the Forgiving, the Merciful."

(Az Zumar 39:53, interpretation of the meaning)

$$\text{قُلْ إِن كُنتُمْ تُحِبُّونَ ٱللَّهَ فَٱتَّبِعُونِى يُحْبِبْكُمُ ٱللَّهُ وَيَغْفِرْ لَكُمْ ذُنُوبَكُمْ ۗ وَٱللَّهُ غَفُورٌ رَّحِيمٌ}$$

Allāh will love you and forgive you your sins; And Allāh is Forgiving and Merciful.

(Ali-Imran 3:31 interpretation of the meaning)

It was narrated from Anas that the Messenger of Allāh (ﷺ)said: "Every son of Adam commits sin, and the best of those who commit sin are those who repent" (Ibn Majah (a)).

Importance of repentance in Islām

Tawbah is a prominent theme in the Qur'ân, mentioned over seventy times, and is the focus of an entire Surah (chapter), *At-Tawbah*:9. Described as turning towards God, seeking forgiveness, and experiencing divine pardon, *tawbah* is a fundamental concept in Islām.

Allāh says in the Qur'ân:

$$\text{وَمَن لَّمْ يَتُبْ فَأُوْلَٰٓئِكَ هُمُ ٱلظَّٰلِمُونَ}$$

And whoever does not repent, it is they who are ⌐true¬ wrongdoers.

(Al-Hujurāt 49:11, interpretation of the meaning)

Ibn Qayyim al Jawziyyah suggested that

> Allāh called the person who did not repent on evildoers. This is because he was the biggest evildoer as he failed to acknowledge his lord and His rights and was not aware of his faults and the bad consequences of his deeds.
>
> (p. 10)

Ibn Qayyim al-Jawziyyah's statement reflects the gravity of failing to repent for one's wrongdoing in Islāmic theology. In Islāmic teachings, repentance is seen as a fundamental aspect of acknowledging one's faults, seeking forgiveness from Allāh, and striving to rectify one's behaviour. By not repenting, a person not only continues in their wrongdoing but also demonstrates a lack of awareness of their own faults and the consequences of their actions. Furthermore, by refusing to repent, an individual may continue to harm themselves and others, perpetuating wrongdoing and contributing to the cycle of sin and disobedience. In essence, by not repenting, one may be considered among the evildoers because they persist in their defiance and disobedience to Allah's guidance. Allāh says in the Qur'ân:

يَـٰٓأَيُّهَا ٱلَّذِينَ ءَامَنُواْ تُوبُوٓاْ إِلَى ٱللَّه تَوۡبَةٗ نَّصُوحًا عَسَىٰ رَبُّكُمۡ أَن يُكَفِّرَ عَنكُمۡ

O you who have believe, repent Allāh with sincere repentance. Perhaps your Lord will remove from you your misdeeds.

(At-Tahrim 66:8, interpretation of the meaning)

إِنَّمَا ٱلتَّوۡبَةُ عَلَى ٱللَّهِ لِلَّذِينَ يَعۡمَلُونَ ٱلسُّوٓءَ بِجَهَٰلَةٖ ثُمَّ يَتُوبُونَ مِن قَرِيبٖ فَأُوْلَـٰئِكَ يَتُوبُ ٱللَّه عَلَيۡهِمۡ وَلَيۡسَتِ ٱلتَّوۡبَةُ لِلَّذِينَ يَعۡمَلُونَ ٱلسَّيِّئَاتِ حَتَّىٰٓ إِذَا حَضَرَ أَحَدَهُمُ ٱلۡمَوۡتُ

The repentance accepted by Allāh is only for those who do wrong in ignorance (or carelessness) and then repent soon after. It is those to whom Allāh will turn in forgiveness, and Allāh is ever Knowing and Wise.
But repentance is not (accepted) of those who [continue to] do evil deeds up until, when death comes to one of them.

(An-Nisa 4:17-18, interpretation of meaning)

The doors of repentance, according to the teachings of Islām, remain open until one's death or until the sun rises from the West (Islām Q&A, 2011). According to Imam An-Nawawi (may Allāh have mercy on him) "Repentance is essential from every sin, even if it is something between a person and Allāh and has nothing to do with the rights of another person" (Islām Q&A, 2011). Al-Agharr bin Yasar Al-Muzani (may Allāh be pleased with him) narrated that: The Messenger of Allāh (ﷺ) said: "Turn you people in repentance to Allāh and beg pardon of Him. I turn to Him in repentance a hundred times a day" (Muslim (a)). This *hadīth* clearly states that sincere repentance means making up for one's mistakes and sins and Allāh accepts the one who repents.

Tawbah is characterised as a dual-purpose technique where individuals are encouraged to both acknowledge their mistakes and actively abandon them in order to seek forgiveness from Allāh. This concept stresses the twofold nature of repentance, emphasising the importance of genuine remorse and a commitment to abandoning sinful behaviour as integral steps in seeking divine forgiveness. The process involves both recognising one's errors and taking proactive measures to rectify them, reflecting a comprehensive approach to spiritual renewal and reconciliation with the divine. Abdullah bin Mas'ud (may Allāh be pleased with him) related to us two narrations: one from the Prophet (ﷺ) and the other from himself, saying: "a believer sees his sins as if he were sitting under a mountain which, he is afraid, may fall on him; whereas the wicked person considers his sins as flies passing over his nose and he just drives them away like this. "Abu Shihab (the sub-narrator) moved his hand over his nose in illustration. (Ibn Mas'ud added): Allāh's Messenger (ﷺ) said, "Allāh is more pleased with the repentance of His slave than a man who encamps at a place where his life is jeopardised, but he has his riding beast carrying his food and water. He then rests his head, sleeps for a short while, and wakes to find his riding beast gone (he starts looking for it) and suffers from severe heat and thirst or what Allāh wished (him to suffer from). He then says, "I will go back to my place." He returns and sleeps again, and then (getting up), he raises his head to find his riding beast standing beside him" (Bukhârî (b)).

On the authority of Anas (may Allāh be pleased with him), who said: I heard the Messenger of Allāh (ﷺ) say: Allāh the Almighty said: O son of Adam, so long as you call upon Me and ask of Me, I shall forgive you for what you have done, and I shall not mind. O son of Adam, were your sins to reach the clouds of the sky and were you then to ask forgiveness of Me, I would forgive you. O son of Adam, were you to come to Me with sins nearly as great as the earth and were you then to face Me, ascribing no partner to Me, I would bring you forgiveness nearly as great as it (Tirmidhî & Ahmad ibn Hanbal). Narrated Abu Sa'id Al-Khudri (may Allāh be pleased with him): The Prophet (ﷺ) said,

> Amongst the men of Bani Israel there was a man who had murdered ninety-nine persons. Then he set out asking (whether his repentance could be accepted or not). He came upon a monk and asked him if his repentance could be accepted. The monk replied in the negative and so

the man killed him. He kept on asking till a man advised to go to such and such village. (So, he left for it) but death overtook him on the way. While dying, he turned his chest towards that village (where he had hoped his repentance would be accepted), and so the angels of mercy and the angels of punishment quarrelled amongst themselves regarding him. Allāh ordered the village (towards which he was going) to come closer to him and ordered the village (whence he had come), to go far away, and then He ordered the angels to measure the distances between his body and the two villages. So, he was found to be one span closer to the village (he was going to). So, he was forgiven.

(Bukhârî (c))

Narrated Ibn Mas`ud (may Allāh be pleased with him): a man kissed a woman (unlawfully) and then went to the Prophet (ﷺ) and informed him. Allāh revealed: and offer prayers perfectly At the two ends of the day And in some hours of the night (i.e. the five compulsory prayers). Verily! good deeds remove (annul) the evil deeds (small sins) (Qur'ân 11.114). The man asked Allāh's Messenger (ﷺ), "Is it for me?" He said, "It is for all my followers." (Bukhârî (d)). Allāh says in the Qur'ân:

$$ إِنَّ ٱلْحَسَنَٰتِ يُذْهِبْنَ ٱلسَّيِّئَاتِ $$

Indeed, good deeds do away with misdeeds.
(Hud 11: 114, interpretation of the meaning)

Anas (may Allāh be pleased with him) reported that a person came to Allāh's Apostle (ﷺ) said: Allāh's Messenger, I have committed an offence which deserves imposition of *haad* [legal or religious punishments, particularly in Islāmic law], so impose it upon me according to the Book of Allāh. Thereupon he said: "Were you not present with us at the time of prayer? He said: Yes. Thereupon he said: You have been granted pardon" (Muslim (b)).

Conditions of repentance

Al-Baghawī, an Islāmic scholar, discussed the differing opinions among scholars regarding the meaning of sincere repentance. Umar and Abu Mu'adh emphasise that it involves repenting and steadfastly avoiding a return to sin, likening it to the irreversible nature of milk leaving the udder. Al-Hasan focuses on the emotional aspect, defining sincere repentance as the regret for past actions coupled with a strong determination to avoid repeating them. Al-Kalbi underlines the multifaceted nature of repentance, involving verbal seeking of forgiveness, profound regret, and self-restraint from wrongful actions. Sa'id ibn Al-Musayyab views sincere repentance as a transformative process that brings tangible benefits to the individual. Al-Qurazi synthesises these elements, proposing a comprehensive definition involving verbal seeking of forgiveness, cessation of sinful actions, internal resolution to avoid repetition, and steering clear of negative influences like bad company. These diverse perspectives collectively contribute to a holistic understanding of sincere repentance in Islāmic thought.

Ibn Qayyim al-Jawziyyah a medieval Islāmic scholar, based his perspective on the conditions of repentance that succinctly captured in three key elements:

- Regret: Sincere repentance involves genuine remorse for one's past actions. This emotional acknowledgement signifies a deep understanding of the wrongdoing and feeling of genuine sorrow for it.
- Desisting: Repentance requires a complete cessation of the sinful behaviour. The repentant individual must actively discontinue the actions and have a firm commitment to abstain from repeating the action in the future.
- Apology: Apologising is not seen as a sign of weakness but rather as a commendable act of humility and sincerity. It is a fundamental aspect of seeking forgiveness from Allāh and fostering harmonious relationships with others. Ibn Qayyim al-Jawziyyah suggested that individual must display both vulnerability and humility, while also showcasing the strength and resilience of the soul.

Al-Makki (1995) suggested 10 conditions in his psychology of *tawbah* (pp. 363–364). The individual is required to cease the sinful behaviour, actively work to avoid committing sins and turn back to God after transgressions. Central to this process is the cultivation of a sincere sense of regret for the wrongdoing, coupled with a commitment to remain upright and avoid future sins. The repentant person should retain a genuine fear of the consequences of their actions while maintaining hope in God's forgiveness. Acknowledging the wrongdoing is essential, as is understanding that God's decree, including the opportunity for repentance, does not diminish His justice. Finally, the process of repentance is completed by following up with righteous acts, serving as a form of repentance for the previous transgressions. This holistic approach reflects the spiritual, emotional, and practical dimensions of seeking forgiveness in Islāmic tradition.

The psychology of *tawbah*

The concept of repentance in Islām involves psychological constructs such as sins, hope, gratitude, and forgiveness. From a psychological perspective, an individual's decision to disclose or withhold their sins is influenced by their beliefs and practices, as well as their perceptions of the implications of the sin. Acknowledging sins is a key aspect of repentance, leading individuals to grapple with feelings of guilt or remorse. Repentance is closely tied to hope, as individuals disclose sins in anticipation of forgiveness and positive transformation. Gratitude plays a role in the repentance process, with individuals expressing thanks for the opportunity to seek forgiveness and rectify their actions. The anticipation of forgiveness serves as a motivating factor, influencing the decision to disclose sins and attain spiritual purification. The psychological dynamics of repentance reflect a complex interplay of emotions, motivations, and spiritual aspirations within the Islāmic framework.

From a psychological perspective, one notable aspect is its function as a cathartic process, allowing individuals to openly express remorse and regret. In essence, catharsis as a form of ventilation of feelings acknowledges the importance of expressing emotions in a healthy and constructive manner. It can contribute to emotional well-being by preventing the accumulation of negative emotions and promoting a more balanced and resilient psychological state. Seeking forgiveness becomes a powerful source of emotional release, alleviating guilt and contributing to emotional well-being. Additionally, *tawbah* instils a sense of responsibility and accountability, as individuals take ownership of their mistakes and actively seek forgiveness. This acknowledgement fosters personal responsibility, contributing to a healthier psychological state.

Furthermore, *tawbah* serves as a motivator for positive change, emphasising the commitment to breaking away from addiction and avoiding its repetition. This resolution becomes a catalyst for personal growth and positive transformation, providing a pathway towards a more virtuous and fulfilling life. The practice also addresses cognitive dissonance by aligning behaviour with moral principles, reducing internal conflicts. The belief in divine forgiveness inherent in *tawbah* instils hope and optimism, promoting resilience and a sense of renewal. Socially, seeking forgiveness from others fosters community support, essential for psychological well-being. Finally, tawbah is deeply intertwined with the purification of the soul (*Tazkiyah an-Nafs*).

Tawbah and the process of change

From a psychological perspective, the TTM (Prochaska et al., 1992, Prochaska & Velicer, 1997) is an integrative model that views behavioural change as a process involving various stages of motivation. The model outlines a series of stages through which individuals progress as they strive to modify their behaviour. The key stages in the TTM are depicted in Figure 6.1. The process of repentance and behaviour change is depicted

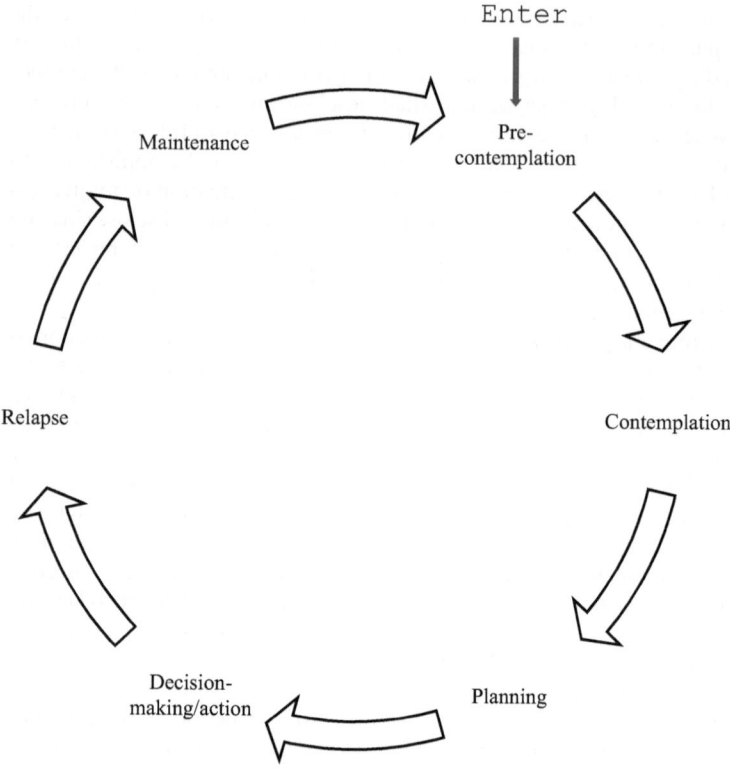

Figure 6.1 Transtheoretical model of change.

through several stages, paralleling the TTM. The initial stage, pre-contemplation, involves individuals in denial about committing sins, lacking recognition of their wrongdoing and awareness of consequences. In the contemplation stage, recognition of sins deepens, fostering true remorse and awareness of the potential benefits of repentance. During preparation, individuals actively ready themselves for seeking forgiveness. And make a resolution to abandon the addiction. The action stage signifies complete repentance to God, employing spiritual strategies to compensate for misdeeds and modifying lifestyles and behaviours. Maintenance progresses, requiring a commitment to uphold changed behaviour and avoid relapse. Relapse is acknowledged as a possible return to sinful behaviour, highlighting the cyclical nature of the repentance process.

At an individual level, the first step to be taken on the path to recovery is to be sincere and to repent. For a Muslim, the doors of repentance are open until you die or until the sun rises from the West It was narrated from Safwan bin 'Assal (may Allāh be pleased with him) that the Messenger of Allāh (☸) said:

> Towards the west (i.e., the place of the setting of the sun) there is an open door, seventy years wide. That door will remain open for repentance until the sun rises from this direction." (Ibn Majah. (b)). Rassool (2021) suggested that "the process of change, in the Islāmic context for *tawbah*, is achieved through the facilitation of five sequential 'movements': identification of the sin or misdeed; de-escalation of the sin or misdeed; making sincere repentance; and re-engagement with the resolution to change and implementing the change; and maintenance of the change.

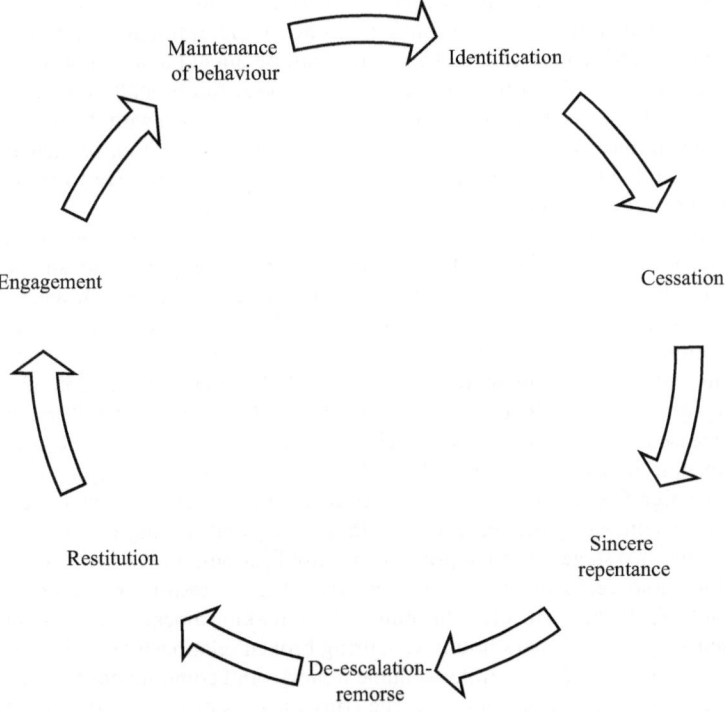

Figure 6.2 Process of change in *tawbah*.

This model has now been modified to include seven sequential "movements" identification, cessation sincere repentance, de-escalation-remorse, restitution, engagement, and maintenance of behaviour (see Figure 6.2).

The second stage of cessation, or *iqla'*, in the process of repentance involves moving beyond mere regret and taking immediate action to stop the sinful behaviour. It requires a decisive and firm commitment to discontinue harmful actions in the present and a pledge to avoid such behaviours in the future. The emphasis is on not only acknowledging the wrongdoing of addiction but also actively and decisively putting an end to the sinful conduct. This stage is accompanied with having the regret to do this. It was narrated that Ibn Ma'qil (may Allāh be pleased with him) said: "I entered with my father upon 'Abdullah, and I heard him say: 'The messenger of Allāh (ﷺ)said: "Regret is repentance." My father said: 'Did you hear the Prophet (ﷺ) say: "Regret is repentance?" He said: 'Yes'" (Ibn Majah (c)). Repentance is accompanied with making ablution and praying *Salaat al-tawbah*, the prayer of repentance, which consists of two Rak'as (units of prayers). This practice is based on the *hādīth* of Abu Bakr al-Siddeeq (may Allāh be pleased with him) and is meant to be performed individually, as it is considered one of the optional prayers not prescribed for congregation. This prayer can be offered at any time, even during periods when other prayers are disallowed. Additionally, engaging in good deeds, such as acts of charity, is encouraged along with the prayer of repentance. While there is no specific guidance on reciting particular Surahs (chapters) during these two Rak'as, individuals are free to recite any portion of the Qur'ân as they see fit (Islām Q&A, 2007).

In the context of the repentance process, de-escalation refers to a behaviour aimed at intensifying feelings of remorse, guilt, and shame (Rassool, 2021). This stage prompts individuals to take specific measures to prevent the repetition of transgressions and involves developing a pure intention. The de-escalation phase is crucial for instilling a heightened sense of commitment to positive change. Following de-escalation, the engagement stage focuses on seeking forgiveness from God through increased supplication, active seeking of forgiveness *(istighfar)*, and engaging in good deeds and charitable activities such as *sadaqah*. This stage signifies a deeper and more sincere commitment to repentance. Openly confessing the sin to God with humility and seeking His pardon signifies this stage. Through prayers and supplications, one expresses contrition and seeks divine mercy. The next stage is restitution (*radd al-maghlub*). If the sin involved harming others, making amends and seeking their forgiveness is paramount. Repairing broken relationships and rectifying the wrong demonstrates genuine remorse and commitment to healing. In the context of addiction, the consequences often extend beyond the individual to impact family and social relationships, leading to significant harm and broken connections with loved ones.

The subsequent maintenance phase ensures the continuity of the newly adopted behaviour, free from past transgressions. This maintenance involves the purification of the soul, known as *Tazkiyah al-Nafs*, which aims to cleanse the heart of vices and immoral behaviours. It encompasses the development of ethical intelligence and the pursuit of moral goodness, ultimately contributing to eternal happiness and overall well-being (*falaḥ*). The maintenance phase underlines the ongoing effort required to uphold positive changes and cultivate a virtuous and purified inner self (Rassool, 2021, pp. 107–108). During this phase, individuals engage in continuous supplications and prayers, seeking God's guidance and strength to resist future temptations and stay on the righteous path. The stage of supplication for protection, or *du'ah*, signifies an acknowledgement of one's vulnerability in the face of temptations and challenges. The act of supplication reflects the recognition that personal strength alone may be insufficient, and it emphasises the spiritual aspect of seeking protection and guidance from Allāh.

Imam Ibn al-Qayyim al-Jazwiyyah stated, "The heart is like a bird; Love is the head, and the two wings are hope and fear." This statement is about the love of Allāh, along with fear of His punishment and hope in His mercy. Abu Hurayrah (may Allāh be pleased with him) narrated that the Prophet (ﷺ) stated:

Allāh Almighty has divided mercy into one hundred parts. He kept ninety-nine parts and sent down one part to earth. Because of that one single part, creatures are merciful to one another so that even the mare will lift its hooves away from its foal so that it does not trample on it.

(Al-Adab Al-Mufrad (b))

The Qur'ān contains more than 112 noble verses which all refer to Allāh Almighty being the "Most Merciful" and this is clear proof that Allāh Almighty's Mercy. Allāh mentions in the Qur'ān:

قُل يَـٰعِبَادِىَ ٱلَّذِينَ أَسْرَفُواْ عَلَىٰ أَنفُسِهِمْ لَا تَقْنَطُواْ مِن رَّحْمَةِ ٱللَّهِ ۚ إِنَّ ٱللَّهَ يَغْفِرُ ٱلذُّنُوبَ جَمِيعًا ۚ إِنَّهُ هُوَ ٱلْغَفُورُ ٱلرَّحِيمُ

Say: O My servants who have transgressed against themselves [by sinning], do not despair of the mercy of Allāh. Indeed, Allāh forgives all sins. Indeed, it is He who is the Forgiving, the Merciful.
(Az-Zumar 39: 53, interpretation of the meaning)

This is how merciful Allāh is. Ibn Kathir (2000) stated:

This ayah [verse] is a call to all sinners, be they disbelievers or others, to repent and turn to Allāh. This ayah tells us that Allāh, may He be blessed and exalted, will forgive all the sins of those who repent to Him and turn back to Him, no matter what or how many his sins are, even if they are like the foam of the sea.

According to the Companion Abdullâh ibn Mas'ood (may Allāh be pleased with him), this is the most hope-inspiring verse of the Qur'ân. Ibn Kathir also maintained that one must not despair of the mercy of Allāh even if one's sins are many and great, for the door of repentance and mercy is expansive. Allāh mentions:

$$وَمَن يَكْسِبْ إِثْمًا فَإِنَّمَا يَكْسِبُهُ عَلَىٰ نَفْسِهِ ۚ وَكَانَ ٱللَّهُ عَلِيمًا حَكِيمًا$$

And whoever does a wrong or wrongs himself but then seeks forgiveness of Allāh will find Allāh Forgiving and Merciful.

(An-Nisa' 4: 110, interpretation of the meaning)

Conclusion

For Muslims dealing with addiction, a comprehensive approach to recovery involves religious, medical, and psychosocial interventions. The process includes sincere repentance (*tawbah*), medical detoxification when appropriate, and psychosocial interventions. Religious support from Islāmic communities, engagement in family therapy, and continued spiritual practices like prayer and Qur'ânic reading are important. Human nature is inherently prone to making mistakes and committing sins. Acknowledging our vulnerability to errors, it becomes essential to engage in a continuous process of repentance and seeking forgiveness. This recognition of our weaknesses highlights the importance of humility, self-reflection, and a commitment to turning back to God whenever we deviate from the righteous path. Repentance serves as a means to reconcile with the Divine, seeking forgiveness for transgressions, and striving for spiritual growth. The cyclical nature of repentance reflects the ongoing journey of self-improvement, emphasising the need for resilience, sincere remorse, and a reliance on divine mercy. Through this perpetual process, individuals can aspire to lead lives aligned with ethical principles and spiritual well-being.

References

Al-Adab Al-Mufrad (a). *Excellence in Character 2302930*. Arabic/English book reference: Book 14, Hādīth 295. Sahih (Al-Albani). https://sunnah.com/urn/2302930

Al-Adab Al-Mufrad (b). Chapter: Mercy consists of a hundred parts 100. *In-book reference: Book 5, Hādīth 17. English translation: Book 5, Hādīth 100.* Sahih (Al-Albani). https://sunnah.com/adab:100

Al-Baghawī. *Tafsīr al-Baghawī (Ma'ā lim al-Tanzīl)* 8/169. Cited in Islām Q&A (2023). Conditions of Repentance. https://Islāmqa.info/en/ answers/289765/conditions-of-repentance, (accessed 21 January 2024).

Al-Makki (1995). Abu Tâlib al-Makki, in Said Nasib (Ed.), *Makrim's Qut al-qulub fi mualamat al mahbub wa-wasf tariq al murid ila maqam al-tawhid.* Beirut: Dar Sadir.

Basiony, D. M. (2017). Your Tawbah (repentance) to-do list: Action points for a fresh start. Repentance... for us! https://productivemuslim. com/tawbah-to-do-list/, (accessed 27 September 2024).

Bukhârî (a). *Sahih al- Bukhârî 5269.* In-book reference : Book 68, Hādīth 19. USC-MSA web (English) reference: Vol. 7, Book 63, Hādīth 194. https://sunnah.com/bukhari:5269#!

Bukhârî (b). *Sahih al- Bukhârî* 6308.In-book reference: Book 80, Hādīth 5. USC-MSA web (English) reference: Vol. 8, Book 75, Hādīth 320. https://sunnah.com/bukhari:6308

Bukhârî (c). *Sahih al- Bukhârî 3470.* In-book reference: Book 60, Hādīth 137. USC-MSA web (English) reference: Vol. 4, Book 55, Hādīth 676. https://sunnah.com/bukhari:3470

Bukhârî (d). *Sahih al- Bukhârî* 526. In-book reference: Book 9, Hādīth 5. USC-MSA web (English) reference: Vol. 1, Book 10, Hādīth 504. https://sunnah.com/bukhari:526

Ibn Kathir. (2000). *Tafsir ibn Kathir*, translated by J. Abualrub, N. Khitab, H. Khitab, A. Walker, M. Al-Jibali, & S. Ayoub. Saudi Arabia: Darussalam Publishers and Distributors.

Ibn Majah (a). *Sunan Ibn Majah 4251.*In-book reference: Book 37, Hādīth 152 English translation: Vol. 5, Book 37, Hādīth 4251. Hasan (Darussalam). https://sunnah.com/ibnmajah:4251

Ibn Majah (b). *Sunan Ibn Majah 4070.* In-book reference: Book 36, Hādīth 145. English translation: Vol. 5, Book 36, Hādīth 4070. Sahih (Darussalam). https://sunnah.com/ibnmajah:4070

Ibn Majah (c). *Sunan Ibn Majah 4252.* Repentance. In-book reference: Book 37, Hādīth 153. English translation: Vol. 5, Book 37, Hādīth 4252. https://sunnah.com/ibnmajah:4252

Ibn Qayyim al Jazwiyyah. *Tawbah: Turing to Allāh in repentance.* Darussalam International Publications Limited. https://www.bing. com/search?q=++Ibn+Qayyim+al-Jawziyya+on+Tawbah&qs=n& form=QBRE&sp=-1&ghc=1&lq=+0&pq=++ibn+qayyim+al-jawziyya+on+tawbah&sc=4-33&sk=&cvi

Islām Q&A. (2007). *Salaat al-tawbah (the prayer of repentance).* https:// Islāmqa.info/en/answers/98030/salaat-al-tawbah-the-prayer-of-repentance, (accessed 21 January 2021).

Islām Q&A. (2011). *Acceptance of repentance.* Fatwa 46683. https:// Islāmqa.info/en/answers/46683/acceptance-of-repentance, (accessed 20 January 2024).

Muslim (a). *Riyad as-Salihin 14. The Book of Miscellany.* Arabic/English book reference: Book 1, Hādīth 14. https://sunnah.com/riyadussalihin:14

Muslim (b). *Sahih Islāmic 2764.* In-book reference: Book 50, Hādīth 52. USC-MSA web (English) reference: Book 37, Hādīth 6660. https:// sunnah.com/Islāmic:2764

Prochaska, J. O., DiClemente, C. C., & Norcross, J. C. (1992). In search of how people change. *American Psychologist*, 47(9), 1102–1114.

Prochaska, J. O., & Velicer, W. K. (1997). The trans-theoretical model of health behaviour change. *American Journal of Health Promotion*, 12(1), 38–48.

Rassool, G. Hussein. (2021). Sins, *Tawbah* and the process of change. *International Journal of Islāmic Psychology*, 4(1), 26–33.

Rassool, G. Hussein. (2023). *Islāmic psychology: The basics*. Oxford: Routledge.

Tirmidhî. *Jami` at-Tirmidhî 3334*. In-book reference: Book 47, Hādīth 386. English translation: Vol. 5, Book 44, Hādīth 3334. Hasan (Darussalam). https://sunnah.com/tirmidhi:3334

7 Spiritual healing

An Islāmic perspective on addressing addiction

Introduction

In recent years, there has been a notable increase in the study of religion and addiction (Faigin et al., 2014; Grubbs et al., 2017; Stauner et al., 2019). The terminology of "Sustained recovery" has been used in the context of addiction which is linked to the concept of 'recovery capital." Recovery capital has been defined as internal and external resources that individuals with addictive disorders can utilise for long-term recovery include peer-based and religious or culturally relevant support groups (UNDOC, 2017). Thus, providing to those who are addicted an enriched spiritual orientation, aiding in the discovery of "meaning and purpose in life." This spiritual connection enhances recovery resources for individuals with addictive behaviours sustaining their capacity to endure long-term recovery from addiction.

Galanter et al. (2021) have proposed an assessment should be undertaken to understand the role of spirituality in their personal history of individuals with addictive disorders. Treatment planning should be informed by an awareness of integrating spiritual considerations to enhance the client's recovery capital. This approach involves examining the client's past experiences with spirituality, identifying relevant spiritual resources in their community, and incorporating suitable community-based resources like culturally oriented facilities, religious institutions, and peer support groups into the client's recovery plan through referrals. "Spiritual Healing: An Islāmic Perspective on Addressing Addiction" explores how Islāmic principles and spirituality contribute to the process of overcoming addiction. This perspective emphasises the significance of spirituality in the recovery journey, aligning with Islāmic teachings and values. The Islāmic perspective on addiction underlines the importance of a holistic approach that encompasses both spiritual and clinical elements, offering insights and guidance for those navigating the challenging path of recovery within an Islāmic framework.

DOI: 10.4324/9781032669212-7

Spiritual capital in addiction recovery

The integration of spirituality in addiction recovery holds paramount importance for Muslim clients, aligning with a holistic approach that addresses the spiritual needs of individuals alongside physical, social and mental dimensions. In Islām, the treatment of addiction extends beyond the body and mind to encompass the soul, emphasising detoxification of the soul as a crucial starting point for recovery and a return to the *fitrah* – the pristine human nature rooted in the belief in the oneness of God. The *fitrah*, intricately woven into various aspects of life, including hope, fear, and overall well-being, serves as a foundation for the recovery process. Reconnecting with Allāh, the Almighty, is seen as pivotal in this process, echoing sentiments expressed by Al-Rāzī in his work "Medicine of the Prophet" (Muḥammad ibn Aḥmad Dhahabī, 1990).

> It is an imperative for every Muslim to draw nearer to God through the offering of righteous deeds, making utmost effort to discharge the divine commands, and showing full obedience. The most effective way leading for that following observing the divine commands and abstinence of prohibitions is what benefits human to keep their health, cure their diseases for seeking the good health is prayers and supplications and acts of worship.
>
> (p.18)

This perspective highlights the significance of spiritual reconnection with God through righteous deeds, strict adherence to divine commands, and complete obedience. Rassool (2021a) introduces the concept of spiritual capital which is referred "as spiritual knowledge, beliefs and practices in accordance with Islāmic theology that is demonstrated in intentional and behavioural actions" (p. 255). Spiritual capital, in the context of addiction, refers to the inherent spiritual resources and strengths available to Muslims engaged in addiction and recovery. This concept recognises the significance of spiritual well-being as a form of capital that individuals can draw upon in their journey towards healing. For Muslims, spiritual capital encompasses a connection to their faith, reliance on Allāh, engagement in spiritual practices, and adherence to Islāmic principles. Spiritual capital is specific to the spiritual and religious domain, where religious practices and beliefs are integral. In contrast, recovery capital is a more inclusive concept that acknowledges a variety of resources, and while it may include spiritual elements for some individuals, it does not dictate a religious component. One basic goal of Islāmic spiritual therapeutic interventions is to purify the soul and strengthen the *taqwa* (God consciousness) will-power, resilience and self-control of the addict. Therapeutic strategies for the Muslim addicts are based on a combination of spiritual, psychosocial and pharmacological approaches in the journey to the recovery process. In a *ḥadīth* narrated on the authority of Abu Hurayrah (may Allāh be pleased with him) that the Messenger of Allāh (ﷺ) said "Allāh does not send down any disease, but He also sends down the cure, except for old age" (Ibn Majah).

Religion can act as a deterrent to alcohol use through several mechanisms, including the influence of positive peer groups, instilling moral values, and enhancing coping skills. Specifically, participation in religious communities may decrease the probability of associating with friends who use alcohol (Koenig et al., 2001). Additionally, Hodge (2011) highlighted that peer groups refraining from alcohol use tend to promote moral values discouraging alcohol consumption.

Principles of Islāmic therapeutic interventions for addiction

Islāmic therapeutic interventions for addicted Muslims are rooted in Islāmic principles and values. Key elements include promoting sincere repentance (*tawbah*), incorporating regular prayers and supplications, remembrance of Allāh, Qur'ânic recitation, *Ruqyah* (incantation), contemplation and Islāmic psychotherapy, and Islāmic-oriented self-help groups and rehabilitation centres. The principles of Islāmic therapeutic interventions for addicted Muslims (Rassool, 2021b) have been modified to include:

- In Islāmic perspective, addiction is recognised as a multifaceted ailment, encompassing spiritual, neurological, and psychosocial dimensions. This view acknowledges the impact of the brain's structure and function alongside spiritual and social factors. Common addictive substances such as alcohol, drugs, tobacco, and gambling are collectively referred to as components of the "Mother of all evils." Despite the severity of addiction, there is a belief in its treatability, emphasising the importance of addressing both the spiritual and physical aspects of the disease within the framework of Islāmic teachings.
- The primary objective in addiction treatment is abstinence. This aligns with the tenets of Islām and the emphasis on abstinence reflects a commitment to a lifestyle free from addictive substances and behavioural addictions.
- Addressing the complex needs of addicted individuals requires comprehensive interventions that go beyond solely focusing on the specific substance use or behavioural addiction. Effectiveness in treatment involves a holistic approach that considers the complex interplay of spiritual, physical, and psychological aspects in the client's life so that broader needs are met to support a comprehensive and sustainable recovery.

- The assessment of a client's needs is an ongoing process, requiring continuous spiritual detoxification and interventions due to the possibility of relapses. In addition to a general assessment, a specific spiritual assessment may be conducted if deemed appropriate. Many individuals struggling with addiction issues often experience co-morbidity, meaning they may also have other psychological disorders such as alcohol dependence and depression. When dealing with Muslim clients presenting with one condition, it is essential to conduct assessments for the presence of other co-occurring disorders to ensure a comprehensive understanding of their mental health needs.
- Effective therapeutic interventions in addressing addiction must align with the holistic needs of the client. Recognising that there is no one-size-fits-all treatment, strategies should be tailored to the specific addiction type, individual personality traits, and the individual's level of *taqwa* (God consciousness) and *Iman* (faith). For muslimwith alcohol and substance se disoder, a comprehensive approach is essential, incorporating bio-psychosocial elements alongside spiritual interventions. While various aspects contribute to the treatment package, the core emphasis lies on providing spiritual guidance and interventions as a central component of the overall therapeutic approach. The treatment package should include comprehensive testing for blood-borne infections and viral diseases such as HIV/AIDS, hepatitis B and C, tuberculosis, COVID-19, and its variants. This testing should be accompanied by pre-test and post-test counselling, along with appropriate treatment measures as needed.
- Detoxification marks the initial phase of addiction treatment, addressing acute physical withdrawal symptoms. However, for Muslims seeking long-term abstinence, sustained recovery requires intensive spiritual interventions beyond detoxification. In addition to spiritual support, pharmacological interventions play a crucial role for many clients and may be integrated as part of harm reduction approaches, when deemed appropriate. Therefore, a comprehensive treatment package for addiction should encompass both spiritual and pharmacological interventions to address the multifaceted nature of the recovery process.
- Psychosocial interventions, when combined with pharmacological approaches, play a vital role in addiction treatment. These interventions encompass various therapeutic modalities such as Islāmic psychotherapy or counselling, cognitive-behavioural therapies, solution-focused therapy, narrative therapy, and humanistic therapy. It is essential that these therapeutic approaches are congruent with Islāmic beliefs and practices, ensuring cultural sensitivity and alignment with the client's faith. Family therapy has shown to enhance family resilience, strengthen family structure, and foster strong familial bonds. Moreover, it has demonstrated improvements in the

problem-solving and coping skills of both the addict and the family, as well as elevated levels of family resiliency (Ulaş & Ekşi, 2019).

- The essence of spiritual interventions is to aid in the purification of the soul, a concept known as *Tazkiyah an Nafs*. This process involves transforming the soul (*nafs*) to cultivate an ideal Muslim personality. The Qur'ân discusses individuals who have purified themselves and emphasises human undertakings in the journey towards refinement. Allāh says in the Qur'ân:

وَمَن تَزَكَّىٰ فَإِنَّمَا يَتَزَكَّىٰ لِنَفْسِهِ

- *And whoever purifies himself only purifies himself for [the benefit of] his soul.* (Fatir 35:18, interpretation of the meaning)
- Incorporating a substantial psychoeducational component into the treatment package is important to ensure that clients understand the potential for relapse despite being on a positive path to recovery. It involves the dissemination of knowledge about addiction, encompassing the consequences of addictive behaviours, factors contributing to recovery, and barriers to healing. A comprehensive psycho-educational programme encompasses the development of social skills, coping skills, assertiveness skills, and relapse prevention strategies. The goal is to empower individuals with the necessary knowledge to prevent relapse and effectively sustain the therapeutic process. Thus emphasising the importance of dealing with the negative consequences of addiction, during the post-detoxification process. The Islāmic psycho-education programme incorporates elements such as prayers, supplications, Qur'ânic study, and aspects of repentance, forgiveness, and gratitude. It emphasises education on the accurate interpretation of belief (*aqeedah*), devotion (*ibadah*), and the practice of virtue, morality, and manners (*akhlaq*) (Alias & Majid, 2005).
- The harm reduction approach is deemed valuable in the treatment package, provided it is appropriate. In the context of the dual challenges posed by alcohol and substance use along with the HIV/AIDS epidemic, harm reduction becomes necessary to safeguard essential elements. In Islāmic legal principles, there exists the provision that allows tolerating a lesser harm to eliminate a greater harm, underlining the pragmatic acceptance of harm reduction as a strategy in addressing the complex issues associated with substance use and health risks.
- It is advisable to match the gender of the therapist with that of the client, prioritising treatment of men by male therapists and women by female therapists. In exceptional circumstances, allowances may be made for necessities that would otherwise be prohibited. Research indicates a preference among female clients for female therapists, supporting the importance of gender concordance in the therapeutic relationship (Fonte & Horton-Deutsch, 2005).

- Addressing the Muslim individual struggling with addiction-related issues involves empowering their soul to fulfil the Divine mission and strengthening adherence to Islāmic principles. It is crucial to remind the client of the Islāmic perspective that during challenging times, Muslims believe that for every hardship, Allāh provides ease. Additionally, emphasising the mercy of Allāh, Muslims understand that facing difficulties can lead to the removal of sins as an act of divine compassion. Allāh says in the Qur'ân:

$$\text{فَإِنَّ مَعَ ٱلْعُسْرِ يُسْرًا}$$
$$\text{إِنَّ مَعَ ٱلْعُسْرِ يُسْرًا}$$

- *For indeed, with hardship [will be] ease [i.e. relief].*
- *Indeed, with hardship [will be] ease.* (Ash-Sharḥ 94:5–6, interpretation of the meaning)

- Clients are encouraged to follow the Islāmic adaptation of the 12 steps from alcoholics anonymous, drug anonymous, or gamblers anonymous as part of their recovery process.
- The client requires support from family, community, and an *Imam*, while maintaining companionship with practising Muslims. The benefits of family involvement include enhancing interpersonal communications and relationships, fostering readiness for change, repairing and strengthening family bonds, overcoming co-dependence or toxic behaviours, providing support to the addict, and learning to establish boundaries for health-oriented behaviours.
- In the addiction recovery process, the *Imam* plays a crucial role in therapy by guiding the client through a re-examination of fundamental Islāmic tenets and promoting behaviours aligned with the Qur'ân and *Sunnah*, as highlighted by Rassool (2016, 2025). Isgandarova (2012) emphasises that Muslim spiritual caregivers aim to facilitate this re-examination process without inducing guilt. Their role is to contribute to the individual's mental and spiritual well-being by fostering a natural balance within the individual and encouraging the practice of social and religious obligations.
- The post-recovery journey for Muslim addicts involves engaging in community services for the *Ummah*, aligning with the four major dimensions supporting recovery according to SAMHSA (2020). Community service is instrumental in sustaining abstinence and self-healing by contributing to meaningful tasks within the community. Volunteering offers opportunities for networking and community support, allowing recovering addicts to restore damaged self-esteem and reintegrate into the real world.
- Overcoming addiction is a prolonged process due to the likelihood of lapses and relapses. Research from the National Institute on Drug Abuse (NIDA) (2018) indicates that most individuals with addiction

require a minimum of three months of treatment to achieve a significant reduction or cessation of drug use. Furthermore, the most favourable outcomes are observed with extended durations of treatment.

* Continuous monitoring of addictive behaviours during therapeutic interventions is essential. This monitoring serves as a potent motivation for addicts to resist urges to use psychoactive substances or engage in gambling activities. Additionally, it provides valuable feedback on the individual's progress in the treatment process.

Islāmic response to alcohol disorder

Badri (2016) criticises Western alcoholism treatments, particularly chemically induced aversion, and defends Islāmic remedies, arguing that they have been misunderstood. He concludes that Muslim therapists should harness the potential power of Islām as a persuasive and aversive force in the treatment of alcoholism. Suliman (1983) recommends a remedy for alcoholism involving a return to "the therapeutic village and the mosque." This suggests that a deeper integration of Muslims into their communities can serve both as a preventive and curative measure for alcoholism. Simultaneously, there is acknowledgement that non-religious therapies for alcoholism may exist and could be combined with Islāmic therapies (Michalak & Trocki, 2006). However, Alias and Majid (2005) emphasise that regardless of the sources of learning, Muslims believe that Allāh is the ultimate reason for learning and behaviour changes. They further note that Islāmic practices such as *wudu`* (ablution), *salat* (prayer), *dhikr* (utterance and remembrance of Allāh), *tilawah* (reading the Qur'ân), and *sawm* (fasting) may contribute positively to preparing for abstinence from alcohol. Additionally, worldly practices such as maintaining a proper diet (semi-vegetarian), using supplements like honey and black seeds (*habbat al-sawda*), and engaging in exercises may also offer positive potentials for behaviour change.

Islāmic response to nicotine and shisha addiction

The majority of *Ahl Sunnah wa'l-Jamaa'ah* scholars have explicitly declared smoking as harām (forbidden). Additionally, the consensus extends to vaping, with a clear stance against it being considered *harām*. In Malaysia, the national fatwa council of the country has officially pronounced e-cigarettes and vaping as harām, reinforcing the prohibition on these practices within an Islāmic context. The Scholars of the Standing Committee issued the following declaration: "Shisha, narghile, and smoking are all evil actions and are haram, because of the harm they cause to one's body and wealth" (Islām Q&A, 2011).

The month of *Ramadan*, known for its emphasis on self-discipline and abstinence, can serve as a powerful incentive for individuals to quit smoking permanently. The heightened spirituality experienced during fasting in *Ramadan* has been suggested to contribute to successful smoking cessation efforts. Studies such as the one conducted by Yong et al. (2009) revealed a significant number of Malaysian Muslims expressing motivation to quit smoking during *Ramadan*. Public health authorities have also utilised the commencement of *Ramadan* as an opportunity to promote and encourage smoking cessation, recognizing the unique motivation and cultural significance of this holy month (Masroor; Ghouri et al., 2006).

The *miswak*, an ancient oral health stick originating from the *Salvadora persica* plant, is being promoted as a helpful aid for smoking cessation during *Ramadan*. Derived from the roots of the plant and known as *arak* in Arabic, the *miswak* is suggested as an alternative to smoking due to its hand-to-mouth action mimicry. Anecdotal evidence supports its use in aiding smoking cessation (Al Sadhan & Almas, 1999) as it mimics the hand to mouth action of people who smoke. Research highlights the oral health benefits of the *miswak*, including antibacterial, antiseptic, anticariogenic, and analgesic properties. Studies comparing it to a toothbrush affirm its efficacy (Dahiya et al., 2012). Additionally, research has explored potential uses beyond oral health, indicating its role as a natural food preservative and a novel functional food ingredient. Overall, the miswak is presented as a potential beneficial tool for those seeking to quit smoking.

Islāmic response to gambling disorder

The Qur'ân addresses drinking and gambling together due to their shared harmful effects on individuals, families, and society. The Islāmic response to gambling mirrors that of alcohol, drug, and tobacco misuse. It emphasises the importance of avoiding gambling and protecting family members. Muslim problem-gamblers are encouraged to seek help from Islāmic psychotherapists and, in some cases, specialist treatment for gambling disorder. The utmost importance is placed on utilising the five daily prayers, supplications, and fasting as beneficial practices for disciplining the soul and seeking protection from *Shaytān*. To address gambling disorders in the context of Islām, harm reduction strategies include increasing awareness through community outreach, educational materials, and workshops. Islāmic psychotherapy and counselling and therapy, particularly cognitive-behavioural therapy, can be provided. Encouraging community support systems, like support groups, helps individuals share experiences and coping strategies. Advocacy for policies and regulations to decrease the availability of gambling opportunities is essential. Additionally, implementing self-exclusion programmes allows individuals to voluntarily ban themselves from gambling venues or online sites.

Islāmic response to cybersex addiction

In addressing cybersex addiction, the therapeutic approach involves recognising the potential utility of abstinence from sexual behaviour as a beneficial technique, although not the primary treatment goal. The overall treatment strategy is centred on gaining control over addictive behaviours and cultivating a healthy approach to sexuality. This includes various interventions such as education on healthy sexuality, Islāmic psychotherapy counselling, marital and family therapy, participation in 12-step programmes, and engagement with self-help groups, as outlined by Rassool (2011). Simultaneously, the Islāmic response to Internet and cybersex addiction integrates spiritual dimensions, emphasising the significance of repentance and seeking support from Allāh. This Islāmic approach advocates acknowledging divine assistance while concurrently endorsing the importance of professional guidance through Islāmic psychotherapy or counselling. The process of seeking repentance and overcoming a sin in Islām involves several steps. It begins with sincere supplication, admission of the sin, and acknowledgment of guilt. The individual is then advised to practice genuine repentance, increase good deeds, and have a sincere intention to cease the sinful behaviour. Contemplation, decision-making, and proactive actions are crucial steps in the process. Continuous remembrance of Allāh (*dhikr*) and supplications are recommended, and if a relapse occurs, the process begins anew. Trusting in Allāh's mercy and maintaining this process until repentance is realized are emphasised throughout.

Islāmic response to pornography addiction

Sound Vision has adapted a set of 12 steps to guide individuals struggling with pornography addiction towards recovery (see Table 7.1). The steps include acknowledging the problem, seeking help, making amends, and incorporating Islāmic principles such as repentance, prayer, and seeking Allāh's guidance. The provided reflection underlines the perceived blessings of Islām's prohibitions and injunctions, highlighting their potential to safeguard individuals and society from the detrimental effects of various addictions. Overall, the adapted steps align with Islāmic teachings, emphasising repentance, seeking support, and incorporating spiritual practices in the journey towards overcoming pornography addiction.

The Family & Youth Institute conducted research in 2022, utilising its findings to create The FYI Porn Addiction Toolkit (Killawi & Rasheed, 2022) which is a comprehensive resource designed to support individuals dealing with porn addiction across three specific areas. The toolkit addresses the needs of those addicted to pornography, spouses of individuals struggling with porn addiction, and parents of children dealing with this issue. It draws on community-based resources to offer tailored

Table 7.1 A 12-step guide to fight pornography addiction

Steps		Actions
1	Admit that you can't give up	Admit that your consumption of pornography is uncontrollable. Every time you turn on the Internet or other media, you cannot say NO to yourself. You cannot abstain from surfing porn sites or stop watching. You are no longer in control of your life.
2	Admit only God can get you out of this	You know that only Allāh can help you out of this due to your inability to abstain from this problem.
3	Your life and death are all in Allāh's control	Put your complete trust in Allāh, who is in control of all aspects of your life and your death. You have chosen to seek His Help first and foremost.
4	You have completed a self-analysis	The painful self-evaluation of your weaknesses and strengths Reflect on your addiction.
5	Made a specific repentance to Allāh	You have admitted to Allāh, to yourself, and to another trusted Muslim (if possible) exactly where you went wrong. You did not make a general request for repentance and listed your mistakes, and in particular, your addiction to pornography.
6	You were open and ready to receive Allāh's help to change	Your repentance to God and sincerity must be followed by action. You are ready to change, no matter how difficult or painful. Even if it means neither watching television for the news or nor surfing the internet alone.
7	You have asked for the removal of faults	You have asked Allāh, with sincerity, humility and regret, to help you to avoid repeating sins committed in the past again.
8	You have decided to seek others' forgiveness	Make a list of everyone you had hurt through your addiction, spouse, children, or parents, and made the intention to approach them seeking forgiveness. You must not, however, disclose your addiction. You just seek forgiveness for any possible act of harm and hurt. Allāh does not like a sin to be advertised.
9	Seek forgiveness from Allāh	Seek the forgiveness and protection of Allāh. Do charity and fast as *kaffārah* if possible.
10	You have completed nightly self-evaluations	Continue self-evaluation of your behaviour and have the readiness to admit your mistakes and thank Allāh for the good you did that day.
11	You have prayed for greater God-consciousness	You prayed and continue to pray five times a day, seeking closeness to Allāh, and have *Taqwa*. Increase your reliance on Him to help you with this addiction to pornography and with all other matters in your life.
12	You preached and practised	Allāh blessed you to get out of this addiction. You helped others with teaching and sincere advice. By the grace of Allāh, helping others helped maintain control over your addiction and helped another person get out of this destruction and misery.

Source: Adapted from Sound Vision (2024).

support and guidance in navigating the challenges associated with porn addiction within these distinct contexts.

Islāmic response to social network addiction

The Islāmic response to Facebook or social network addiction involves a reflective examination of the reasons for joining the platform. Individuals are encouraged to assess their initial motivations, whether for knowledge enrichment, social connection, or other purposes. Narrated Al-Mughira bin Shu`ba (may Allāh be pleased with him): The Messenger of Allāh
(ﷺ) said, "And Allāh has hated for you vain, useless talk, or that you talk too much about others" (Bukhârî). Considering the *hadīth* discouraging vain and useless talk, users are advised to reflect on the purpose of their online interactions. Practical steps include creating an Internet schedule, limiting time online to align with real goals, and turning to Allāh in repentance for support. Seeking Islāmic psychotherapy or counselling and consulting with an Imam are emphasized as additional measures to address and overcome Facebook addiction within the framework of Islāmic principles.

Spiritual healing

Spiritual healing or medicine known as *"al-ṭibb al-ruhī or al-ruhīna"* focuses on the treatment or reformation of the soul through spiritual interventions (Ar-Razi, 1978, pp. 51–52). Allāh says in the Qur'ân:

$$ لا وَنُنَزِّلُ مِنَ ٱلْقُرْءَانِ مَا هُوَ شِفَآءٌ وَرَحْمَةٌ لِّلْمُؤْمِنِينَ $$

And we send down of the Qur'ân that which is healing and mercy for the believers.

(Al-Isra'17: 82, interpretation of the meaning)

For Muslims facing challenges such as alcohol problems, the ultimate path to salvation involves turning to Allāh, reading the Qur'ân, and seeking forgiveness and help. Additionally, it is emphasised that individuals with addiction should actively seek professional treatment. Seeking such treatment aligns with Islāmic principles, and the method of treatment is clearly prescribed within the faith. Jabir (may Allāh be pleased with him) reported Allāh's Messenger (ﷺ) as saying: "There is a remedy for every malady, and when the remedy is applied to the disease it is cured with the permission of Allāh, the Exalted and Glorious" (Muslim (a)). The spiritual interventions include making supplication, remembrance of Allāh, healing from the Qur'ân, prayer as a coping strategy, trust in Allāh (*tawakkul*), and Prophetic medicine (See Rassool, 2021b). In Islām, those who seek treatment are not stigmatised or shamed; rather, the faith encourages an attitude of compassion and support. Islām teaches that illness, whether physical, mental, or spiritual, is a test from Allāh, and seeking healing is a virtuous act. The belief that Allāh is Merciful and Forgiving reassures believers that turning to treatment or support is part of a holistic process of self-care, healing, and faith. he responsibility lies in supporting and assisting in the rehabilitation of individuals whenever possible.

Islāmic-oriented rehabilitation centres

Islāmic-oriented rehabilitation centres, albeit limited, are now available for Muslims grappling with addiction-related issues. Notably, Millati Islāmi, known for its "Path of Peace" 12-step recovery programme in the United States, stands out as a prominent example. Millati Islāmi is designed to address a range of addictions, including those to drugs/alcohol, violence, anger, or food. Millati Islāmi is a "Fellowship of man and women look to Allāh to guide us on Millati Islāmi (the Path of Peace). While recovering, we strive to become rightly guided Muslims, submitted our will and services to Allāh." This recovery support group has adapted the 12 steps to incorporate Islāmic principles in their "Therapy Can Help Overcome Addiction" (www.millatiIslāmi.org). Table 7.2 compares between the 12 steps and Millati Islāmi models.

The Millati Islāmi programme is based on the notions that

* As recovering addicts, we strive to become rightly guided Muslims, submitting our will to the will and service of Allāh.
* We begin the process of submission through the practice of Islam in our daily lives.
* Millati Islāmi strives to equip the individual with the necessary tools of awareness and understanding to break the cycle of addictions.
* Millati Islāmi is also based on the sin model. As taught from the Qur'ân, addictions are a sin, which have a negatively affect an individual's life.
* Within the programme, we follow the Islāmic prophetic example as a route to productive, healthier, and drug-free lives.

The Muslim Recovery Network Programme in Birmingham, UK, and Minds Alive in Durban, South Africa, both offer 12-step recovery programmes grounded in Islāmic principles. In Birmingham, the programme, spanning six weeks, draws inspiration from the Islāmic prophetic example, guiding individuals towards productive, healthier, and drug-free lives. It encourages exploration of addiction and emphasises the role of religious and spiritual healing in achieving successful recovery. Minds Alive in

Table 7.2 Comparison between the twelve steps and Millati Islāmi models

The 12 steps model	*Millati Islāmi**
Admitted we were powerless over alcohol; that our lives had become unmanageable;	We admit that we are powerless over drugs and that our lives have become unmanageable.
Came to believe that a Power greater than ourselves could restore us to sanity;	We have come to believe that Allāh can restore us to sanity.
Made a decision to turn our will and our lives over to the care of God as we understood Him;	We have made a decision to turn our wills and our lives over to the care of Allāh.
Made a searching and fearless moral inventory of ourselves;	We have made a searching and fearless moral inventory of ourselves in the light of the Islāmic doctrines (*Shar'iah*).
Admitted to God, to ourselves, and to another human being the exact nature of our wrongs;	We admit to Allāh and to ourselves the exact nature of our wrongs.
Were entirely ready to have God remove all these defects of character;	We are entirely ready to pray to Allāh to remove all these defects of character.
Humbly asked Him to remove our shortcomings;	We have humbly asked Him to remove our shortcomings.
Made a list of all persons we had harmed and became willing to make amends to them all;	We have made a list of all persons we have harmed, and we have become willing to make amends to all.
Made direct amends to such people wherever possible, except where to do so would injure them or others;	We have made direct amends to such people wherever possible, except when to do so would injure them or others.
Continued to take a personal inventory and, when we were wrong, promptly admitted it;	We continue to take personal inventory and, when we do wrong, we promptly admit it.
Sought through prayer and meditation to improve our conscious contact with God as we understood Him, praying only for knowledge of His will for us and the power to carry that out;	We seek through prayer and other religious commitments and activities to improve our conscious contact with Allāh, praying only for knowledge of His will for us and the power to carry that out.
Having had a spiritual experience (awakening) as the result of these steps, we tried to carry this message to alcoholics, and to practise these principles in all our affairs.	We have had a spiritual awakening as the result of these steps. We try to carry this message to problem drug users and practise these principles in all our affairs.

* *Source*: Adapted from Salem and Ali (2008).

Durban is founded on the idea that avoiding addiction prompts reflection on the reality of death and the meaning of life. Through remembrance of Allāh and seeking His pleasure, Muslim addicts are motivated and inspired to overcome addiction, aligning with Islāmic principles for a holistic approach to recovery.

Ibn al-Qayyim al-Jawziyyah identified two major categories psychoeducation and behavioural instruction in the management and treatment of those with addiction (Abdul-Rahman, 2023). He also developed 50 strategies for treating addiction (Ibn al-Qayyim, 2010). Under the categorisation of psychoeducation, Ibn al-Qayyim addresses both the negative consequences of addiction and the positive outcomes of healing, reinforcing the motivation for change. Additionally, he outlines positive qualities integral to the healing journey, such as sincerity, courage, and patience, which need cultivation. According to Ibn al-Qayyim, addiction serves as a starting point for ethical and spiritual transformation, with negative qualities identified as barriers to healing that must be overcome during the rehabilitation process (Abdul-Rahman, 2023). Behavioural instruction, as discussed by Ibn al-Qayyim, revolves around the intriguing theme of visualisation, which aligns with guided imagery therapy – an approach recently evaluated for addiction treatment. Guided imagery therapy aims to induce positive changes in thoughts and behaviours while alleviating symptoms of mental illness and enhancing coping skills. This therapeutic modality encompasses various techniques, including the "reinstatement of dream image," which involves actual dreams, fantasies, or daydreams. The application of visualisation in addiction treatment highlights the relevance of his insights in addressing addiction and promoting holistic well-being.

Ibn al-Qayyim (2010) develop a psychospiritual programme in the rehabilitation addicts. This is depicted in Figure 7.1. Abdul-Rahman (2023) discusses Ibn al-Qayyim's five-step rehabilitation programme for overcoming addiction. This revolves around a systematic and holistic approach, emphasising the importance of psycho-spiritual development. Ibn al-Qayyim encourages individuals struggling with addiction to actively seek knowledge and contemplate the consequences of surrendering to forbidden desires. This process of learning serves as a catalyst, fostering heightened motivation to overcome those desires and instilling a profound aversion to succumbing to failure. This psycho-spiritual state, characterised by increased awareness and determination, marks the initial step towards the journey of recovery. Reconnection with the concept of *tawḥīd* (Islāmic monotheism) is advocated and achieved through practices like Qur'ân recitation, contemplation of scripture, studying prophetic traditions, and gaining beneficial knowledge. The individual is then guided to purify their environment [personal and social], safeguarding against potential triggers or cues and actively protecting themselves from negative influences or desires. Spiritual hygiene, seeking refuge in Allāh, and contemplation in daily activities contribute to maintaining a virtuous lifestyle. The programme stresses the development of patience *(ṣabr)* through positive actions, balanced rest, and proper time management. During periods free from impulses, individuals implement these lifestyle changes, and when cravings arise, prescribed visualisations and guided imagery are employed to offset impulsive behaviour.

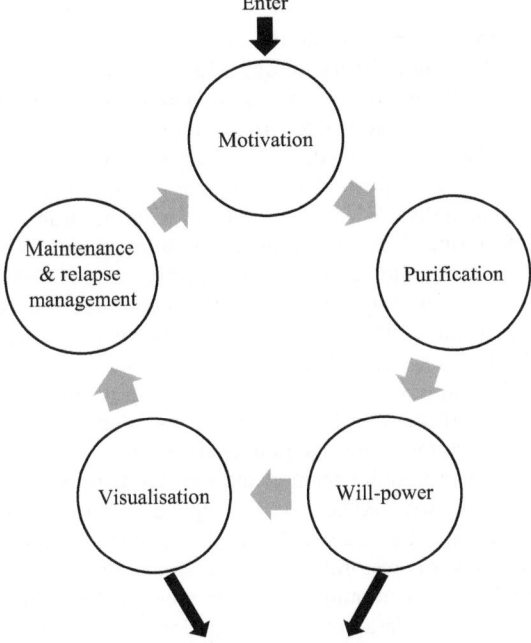

Exit & re-enter at any stage

Source: Adapted from Abdul-Rahman (2023)

Figure 7.1 Ibn Qayyim's five-step rehabilitation programme for addiction.

Overall, the narrative highlights a comprehensive approach integrating motivation, spiritual practices, environmental awareness, and psychological techniques to guide individuals on the path to recovery.

While literature on government rehabilitation centres for addiction recovery is limited, there is a prevalence of private hospitals and clinics addressing the treatment and rehabilitation needs of Muslim struggling with alcohol and substance use disorder. These facilities extend beyond Tehran, Iran, to encompass hospitals in the Kingdom of Saudi Arabia, government-run drug and alcohol rehabilitation centres in the UAE, and recovery support groups such as alcoholics anonymous (AA) and narcotics anonymous (NA) in Dubai. Significant examples include Hayat House in Sydney, Australia, offering culturally appropriate, community-based rehabilitation for Muslim individuals struggling with drug and alcohol addiction. Globally, there are faith-based treatment centres with services tailored for addicted Muslims, often accompanied by the availability of religious advisors for spiritual counselling and healing.

Conclusion

The chapter focuses on the profound impact of integrating Islāmic spirituality into addiction recovery among Muslims. It highlights the significance of spiritual capital, encompassing Islāmic knowledge, beliefs, and practices, as an important asset in the journey towards healing from addiction. Islāmic therapeutic interventions advocate for holistic approaches that blend spiritual, psychosocial, and pharmacological methods tailored to individual needs. By facilitating spiritual reconnection with God, fostering sincere repentance, and offering comprehensive psychoeducation, these interventions aim to purify the soul and fortify resilience. Islāmic responses to addiction reveal a complex understanding of the intricate dynamics between spiritual well-being, psychological health, and social support systems. The incorporation of Islāmic principles into therapeutic modalities provides comprehensive frameworks for addressing addiction challenges. Insights derived from Islāmic perspectives offer valuable guidance for clinicians, policymakers, and communities in nurturing resilience, promoting healing, and facilitating recovery among individuals grappling with addiction. Through collaborative undertakings grounded in compassion and faith-based principles, Islāmic approaches pave the way towards restoration, renewal, and transformation for individuals, families, and communities alike in their challenges tacking addictive behaviours. Islamic approaches to addressing addictive behaviours pave the way for restoration, renewal, and transformation for individuals, families, and communities. By emphasising collaborative efforts rooted in compassion and faith-based principles, these approaches foster healing and positive change. They provide holistic support systems that address the complex needs of individuals grappling with addiction, ultimately leading to improved well-being and resilience at the personal, familial, and community levels.

References

Abdul-Rahman, Z. (2023). *How to overcome addiction through faith: Ibn-Qayyim's rehabilitation programme*. Irving, TX: Yaqeen Institute.

Al Sadhan, R. I., & Almas, K. (1999). Miswak (chewing stick): A cultural and scientific heritage. *Saudi Dental Journal*, 11(2), 80–88.

Alias, A., & Majid, H. S. A. (2005). Psychology of learning from an Islāmic perspective. Presented at the *3rd International Seminar on Learning and Motivation* (10–12 September 2005) organised by Faculty of Cognitive Sciences & Education Universiti Utara Malaysia at City Bayview Hotel, Langkawi, Kedah, Malaysia.

Ar-Razi, F. (1978). *At-Thibb Ar-Ruhani*. Cairo: Maktabat al-Nahda al-Misriyya.

Badri, M. (2016). *The dilemma of Muslim psychologists*. Kuala Lumpur: Islamic Book Trust.

Bukhârî. *Sahih al- Bukhârî 2408*. In-book reference: Book 43, Hadith 23. USC-MSA web (English) reference: Vol. 3, Book 41, Hadith 591. https://sunnah.com/bukhari:2408

Dahiya, P., Kamal, R., Luthra, R. P., Mishra, R., & Saini, G. (2012). Miswak: A periodontist's perspective. *Journal of Ayurveda and Integrative Medicine*, 3(4), 184–187.

Faigin, C. A., Pargament, K. I., & Abu-Raiya, H. (2014). Spiritual struggles as a possible risk factor for addictive behaviors: An initial empirical investigation. *The International Journal for the Psychology of Religion*, 24(3), 201–214. https://doi.org/10.1080/10508619.2013.837661

Fonte, J., & Horton-Deutsch, S. (2005). Treating postpartum depression in immigrant Muslim women. *Journal of the American Psychiatric Nurses Association*, 11(1), 39–44.

Galanter, M., Hansen, H., & Potenza, N. (2021). The role of spirituality in addiction medicine: A position statement from the spirituality interest group of the international society of addiction medicine. *Substance Abuse*, 42(3), 269–271. https://doi.org/10.1080/08897077.2021.1941514

Ghouri, N., Atcha, M., & Sheikh, A. (2006). Influence of Islām on smoking among Muslims. *BMJ (Clinical Research Education)*, 332(7536), 291–294.

Grubbs, J. B., Exline, J. J., Pargament, K. I., Volk, F., & Lindberg, M. J. (2017). Internet pornography use, perceived addiction, and religious/spiritual struggles. *Archives of Sexual Behavior*, 46(6), 1733–1745. https://doi.org/10.1007/s10508-016-0772-9

Hodge, D. R. (2011). Alcohol treatment and cognitive-behavioral therapy: Enhancing effectiveness by incorporating spirituality and religion. *Social Work*, 56(1), 21–31.

Ibn al-Qayyim. (2010). *Rawḍat al-muḥibbīn*, ed. Muḥammad ʿAzīz Shams. Jeddah: Dār ʿAlam al-Fawāʾid.

Ibn Majah. *Sunan Ibn Majah 3436*. In-book reference: Book 31, Hadith 1.English translation: Vol. 4, Book 31, Hadith 3436. Sahih (Darussalam). https://sunnah.com/ibnmajah:3436

Isgandarova, N. (2012). Effectiveness of Islāmic spiritual care: Foundations and practices of Muslim spiritual care givers. *The Journal of Pastoral Care & Counseling: JPCC*, 66(3–4), 4.

Islām Q&A. (2011). *Ruling on smoking the Argileh or Shisha and a discussion on its harmful effects*. Fatwa 127312. https://Islāmqa.info/en/answers/127312/ruling-on-smoking-the-argileh-or-shisha-and-a-discussion-on-its-harmful-effects, (accessed 22 January 2024).

Killawi, I., & Rasheed, M. (2022). *Porn addiction toolkit* https://thefyi.org/porn-addiction-toolkit/, (accessed 22 January 2024).

Koenig, H. G., McCullough, M. E., & Larson, D. B. (2001). *Handbook of religion and health*. New York: Oxford University Press.

Masroor, A. (Ed.). *Ramadan health guide. A guide to healthy fasting*. London: Communities in Action.

Michalak, L., & Trocki, K. (2006). Alcohol and Islam: An overview. *Contemporary Drug Problems*, 33(4), 523-562. https://doi.org/10.1177/009145090603300401

Muḥammad ibn Aḥmad Dhahabī. (1990). *al-Ṭibb al-Nabawī* (3rd ed.), ed. Ahmad Rifʿat al-Badrawi. Beirut: Dar Ihya al-ʿUlum.

Muslim (a). *Sahih Muslim 2204*. In-book reference: Book 39, Hadith 95. USC-MSA web (English) reference: Book 26, Hadith 5466. https://sunnah.com/muslim:2204

National Institute on Drug Abuse (NIDA). (2018). *Principles of drug addiction treatment: A research-based guide* (3rd ed.). https://nida.nih.gov/sites/default/files/podat-3rdEd-508.pdf#:~:text=This%20update%20of%20the%20National%20Institute, (accessed 27 September 2024).

National Institute on Drug Abuse (NIDA). (2020). *Principles of effective treatment. A research based guide.* https://www.drugabuse.gov/download/675/principles..., (accessed 22 January 2024).

Rassool, G. Hussein. (2011). *Understanding addiction behaviours: Theoretical & clinical practice in health and social care.* Basingstoke, Hampshire: Palgrave McMillan.

Rassool, G. Hussein. (2016). *Islāmic counselling. An introduction to theory and practice* (Ist ed.). Hove, Sussex: Routledge.

Rassool, G. Hussein. (2021a). *Islāmic psychology: human behaviour and experience from an Islāmic perspective.* Oxford: Routledge.

Rassool, G. Hussein. (2021b). *Mother of all evils: Addictive behaviours from an Islāmic perspective.* Islāmic Psychology Publishing (IPP) & Institute of Islāmic psychology Research (IIPR). Amazon/Kindle.

Rassool, G. Hussein. (2025). *Islāmic counselling & psychotherapy* (2nd ed.). Oxford: Routledge.

Richards, P. S., & Potts, R. W. (1995). Using spiritual interventions in psychotherapy: Practices, successes, failures, and ethical concerns of Mormon psychotherapists. *Professional Psychology: Research and Practice*, 26(2), 163–170. https://doi.org/10.1037/0735-7028.26.2.163

Salem, M.O., & Ali, M. (2008). Psycho-spiritual strategies in treating addiction patients: Experience at Al-Amal Hospital, Saudi Arabia. *Journal of the Islamic Medical Association of North America*, 40.

SAMHSA. (2020). *Recovery and recovery support.* Rockville, MD: Substance Abuse and Mental Health Services Administration. https://www.samhsa.gov/find-help/recovery, (accessed 22 January 2024).

Sound Vision. (2024). *A 12-step guide to fight pornography addiction.* https://www.soundvision.com/article/a-12-step-guide-to-fight-pornography-addiction, (accessed 22 January 2024).

Stauner, N., Exline, J. J., Kusina, J. R., & Pargament, K. I. (2019). Religious and spiritual struggles, religiousness, and alcohol problems among undergraduates. *Journal of Prevention & Intervention in the Community*, 47(3), 243–258. https://doi.org/10.1080/10852352.2019.1603678

Suliman, H. (1983). Alcohol and Islāmic faith. *Drug and Alcohol Dependence*, 11(1), 63–65.

The Family & Youth Institute. (2022). *Pornography & Muslim youth: Preliminary research findings*. https://thefyi.org/pornography-muslim-youth-preliminary-research-findings/, (accessed 22 January 2024).

Ulaş, E., & Ekşi, H. (2019). Inclusion of family therapy in rehabilitation program of substance abuse and its efficacious implementation. *The Family Journal*,27(4),443–451.https://doi.org/10.1177/1066480719871968

United Nations Office on Drugs and Crime (UNDOC). (2017). *International standards for the treatment of drug use disorders 2017*. Geneva. World Health Organization. https://www.who.int/substance_abuse/activities/msb_treatment_standards.pdf, (accessed 21 January 2024).

www.millatiislami.org. http://www.millatiislami.org/Welcome/12-steps, (accessed 22 January 2024).

Yong, H. H., Hamann, S. L., Borland, R., Fong, G. T., Omar, M., & ITC-SEA Project Team (2009). Adult smokers' perception of the role of religion and religious leadership on smoking and association with quitting: A comparison between Thai Buddhists and Malaysian Muslims. *Social Science & Medicine*, 69(7), 1025–1031.

Index

Page numbers in **bold** refer to tables.